# Drugs and Appetite

# Drugs and Appetite

*edited by*

## T. Silverstone

*Academic Unit of Human Psychopharmacology*
*Medical College of St. Bartholomew's Hospital, London*

1982

## ACADEMIC PRESS

*A Subsidiary of Harcourt Brace Jovanovich, Publishers*

London   New York
Paris   San Diego   San Francisco
São Paulo   Sydney   Tokyo   Toronto

ACADEMIC PRESS INC. (LONDON) LTD.
24/28 Oval Road
London NW1

*United States Edition published by*
ACADEMIC PRESS INC.
111 Fifth Avenue
New York, New York 10003

*British Library Cataloguing in Publication Data*

Silverstone, T.
 Drugs and appetite.
 1. Appetite — Physiological aspects
 2. Weight reducing preparations
 I. Title
 612'.3–1     QP147

 ISBN 0–12–643780–7

 LCCCN 81–67903

Phototypesetting by Oxford Publishing Services
Printed in Great Britain by
Thomson Litho Ltd, East Kilbride, Scotland

# ☐ Contributors

J. E. Blundell: *Psychology Department, University of Leeds*

M. J. Ford: *Royal Infirmary, Edinburgh*

S. Garattini: *Instituto di Ricerche Farmacologiche "Mario Negri", Milan*

M. Kyriakides: *Academic Unit of Psychopharmacology, Medical College of St. Bartholomew's Hospital, London*

C. J. Latham: *Psychology Department, Goldsmith's College, University of London*

J. F. Munro: *Eastern General and Edenhall Hospitals and Department of Medicine, Western General Hospital, Edinburgh*

R. Samanin: *Instituto di Ricerche Farmacologiche "Mario Negri", Milan*

T. Silverstone: *Academic Unit of Human Psychopharmacology, Medical College of St. Bartholomew's Hospital, London*

G. P. Smith: *Department of Psychiatry, Cornell University Medical College and Edward W. Bourne Behavioral Research Laboratory, New York Hospital — Cornell Medical Center, White Plains, N.Y.*

G. I. Szmukler: *Academic Department of Psychiatry, Royal Free Hospital and Institute of Psychiatry, London*

# ☐ Preface

The purpose of this monograph is to give a comprehensive and up-to-date account of the ways in which drugs can influence appetite, both in laboratory animals and in human subjects. This should lead to a better understanding of the ways in which such drugs act on physiological mechanisms within the body, and, as a consequence, provide a rational basis for the use of these drugs in clinical practice. Rational prescribing also depends on knowledge of the pharmacological properties of the available drugs. To these ends this book includes chapters on the physiology, the behavioural pharmacology, and the clinical pharmacology of appetite and feeding, plus clinical chapters relating to drug treatment in the management of obesity and anorexia nervosa.

While there is little, if any, disagreement about what drugs are, there is far less consensus concerning the meaning and usage of the term appetite. In his opening chapter on the physiology of feeding, Smith chooses to eschew the term completely, pointing out that it usually refers to feeding in general. He fails to find any value in making a distinction between hunger and appetite, remarking that the concept of hunger, as distinct from appetite, has not helped physiological analysis in any way. Blundell, on the other hand, in his discussion of feeding behaviour in laboratory animals, does distinguish between the two concepts, regarding hunger as a "deficit signal" which primarily influences the onset of eating, while appetite, "is engendered by certain features of the diet, and exerts a primary control over the maintenance of eating".

For my own part, I take a view of these terms which incorporates some of the underlying thinking of both Smith and Blundell. As far as studies in laboratory animals are concerned, I would agree with Smith that to attempt to differentiate, or even to use, the concepts of appetite and hunger can be misleading in such a setting, as all that can be observed directly is feeding behaviour; there is no way of knowing what the animal actually *feels*, we can only see what it *does*. I do believe, however, that these terms have some value when it comes to the study of human subjects. Here I would agree with Blundell in applying the term "hunger" to describe those psychological sensations which accompany significant food deprivation. As I attempt to show in my chapter on the measurement of hunger and food intake in man, the degree to which these sensations are experienced at a given time can be reliably quantified, and are predictable and consistently responsive to pharmacological manipulation. Where I differ from Blundell is in the use of the term "appetite". I regard it as referring to an individual's desire for food, *however brought about*. That is, while physiologically determined hunger can influence appetite to a greater or lesser degree, changes in the desire for food (appetite) can be at least partly independent of hunger. For example, we often respond to the sight or smell of a particular food by eating, even though we may not be particularly hungry at the time. The distinction between appetite and hunger becomes even more evident when we consider the role of emotional and cognitive factors in determining eating behaviour as, for example, occurs in anorexia nervosa.

In spite of such semantic differences there is, nevertheless, general agreement about relating the term "appetite" in some manner to feeding. In this volume we are concerned with describing how drugs interact with appetite, and hence with feeding behaviour, and how such interaction can in turn lead to changes in body weight, the goal of most treatment programmes directed towards the clinical problems of obesity and anorexia nervosa.

Before we can begin to understand the pharmacological mechanisms by which drugs exert their influence on feeding and appetite, we need to know the physiological processes by which feeding behaviour is normally regulated. In his opening chapter entitled "The Physiology of the Meal", Smith emphasizes that the functional unit of feeding in virtually all mammalian species is the meal. In order to understand the physiology of meal eating behaviour, he regards it as sensible to consider in turn the factors which appear to influence the beginning and ending of a meal, together with the pattern of ingestion observed during the meal. Setting about his task in a manner refreshingly free from any theoretical preconceptions, he provides a most scholarly account of the integrated physiological events which influence meal eating behaviour. His analysis is truly Sherringtonian in scope.

Samanin and Garattini have chosen to consider the basic neuropharmacology of the currently available appetite suppressants from the standpoint of their actions on certain neurotransmitter systems of the brain, namely the noradrenergic, dopaminergic and serotonergic pathways. They show how anorectic compounds and specific receptor-blocking drugs can be used as scalpels with which to dissect out the various components within the brain which influence feeding. We shall see later how such insights into the neuropharmacological action of appetite-suppressant (i.e. anorectic) drugs in laboratory animals can provide the impetus for parallel experiments in man.

Blundell, in his chapter on the behavioural pharmacology of feeding, points out how necessary it is to apply to the study of the behaviour of feeding, the same methodological rigour which underpins the study of its pharmacology. To this end, he describes ways in which the "fine-grain" of feeding behaviour can be examined in detail, and goes on to discuss the sometimes unexpected effects which appetite-suppressant drugs can have on this behaviour. In his most erudite contribution, Blundell draws from a wide range of academic disciplines, nowhere more effectively than when he talks about the "bio-grammar" of feeding, a term he has adopted from the field of linguistics.

In my chapter on the measurement of hunger and food intake in man, I demonstrate how techniques developed in the field of behavioural pharmacology can be adapted for use in human subjects, and it will be evident that our techniques for the measurement of human feeding are derived from the methods originally devised by Blundell to monitor continuous free-feeding behaviour in rats.

Our review of the clinical pharmacology of appetite attempts to relate how concepts developed in neuropharmacological experiments in laboratory animals can be applied to the study of the effect of drugs on human feeding; such an approach can, we believe, assist us to gain further understanding of the possible neural mechanisms underlying this behaviour. In fact, human psychopharmacology in general depends on a continuing dialogue between the student of basic pharmacology and the student of human behaviour: neither alone suffices. For example, as I have already indicated, it is impossible in rats to know what the animal actuallly feels in terms of hunger or emotion; we must turn to human studies for such information. Conversely, it is currently impossible to probe directly into the human nervous system to examine the precise neurochemical changes which a drug may be producing within a specified part of the brain; we depend on studies of animal brains to provide such information. And it is therefore necessary to extrapolate repeatedly from one discipline to the other in order to progress.

The final two chapters are concerned with the clinical applications of drugs in the management of disorders of body weight (which, in the case of obesity at least, does not necessarily imply an underlying disorder of appetite). Certain appetite-suppressant drugs are widely prescribed for the treatment of obesity, and are thought to be of some benefit by a large number of patients. Unfortunately in my view, more time has been spent publicizing the potential disadvantages of drug treatment in obesity than on trying to define its proper place. As Munro and Ford point out in their chapter on drug treatment in obesity, most obese patients do not eat more than their contemporaries; therefore what they need is help in reducing their dietary intake *below the norms of their society*. Furthermore, such dietary restriction, and consequently such assistance, will be required for many months, if not years. This is in sharp contrast to the prevailing conventional wisdom expressed in the view that all obese patients are probably self-indulgent gluttons lacking in will-power; therefore moral exhortation rather than medical treatment is what is required. Sadly this puritanical attitude to the problem has led to irrational, illogical and inconsistent advice about the use of appetite-suppressant drugs in clinical practice. I would, of course, agree with Munro and Ford that such drugs should only be given as an integral part of a dietary programme. But, as they point out, they are effective for only as long as they are taken. That should hardly surprise us, yet one of the arguments which has been levelled at appetite-suppressant drugs is that they do not "re-educate" the patient to eat less; in other words they do not help him eat less when they are no longer being prescribed. To expect such an effect is, in my view, naïve, and smacks of inconsistency; we would not, for example, expect an analgesic drug to relieve the pain of an osteo-arthritic knee beyond the time the drug is being taken.

Anorectic drugs are also castigated for causing dependence, tolerance and abuse, and thus are considered as being dangerous as well as useless. Let us examine each of these concepts in turn. There is no evidence for these drugs causing physical dependence, with consequent withdrawal symptoms, other than in the case of fenfluramine, where sudden withdrawal can lead to depressive symptoms. Nor is there much evidence to support psychological dependence being a significant clinical problem; most patients who are prescribed these drugs have little or no difficulty in stopping them. The fact that they only work when they are being taken can hardly be counted as evidence in favour of dependency-producing propensity.

Tolerance refers to the reduction in clinical response observed with the increasing length of time a particular drug is taken. Certainly the rate of weight loss may fall off with time, but in the clinical trials in which the effects of anorectic drugs have been studied for any length of time, weight loss attributable to the anorectic drug under investigation has continued to exceed that observed in the comparison group of patients receiving inert placebo for as long as the trial has proceeded. Furthermore, the fall in rate of weight loss with time is unlikely to reflect true pharmacological tolerance as we have shown that the rate of weight loss due to an anorectic drug in patients who have already received the drug for the previous month is not appreciably less than that observed in patients receiving the active drug for the first time.

Finally, abuse; this term refers to the self-administration of a substance, taken in greater than therapeutic quantities for non-therapeutic purposes. It rarely occurs in obese patients: the abuse of appetite-suppressant drugs for their stimulant effect is largely confined to teenagers and young adults who have no weight problem, and who have most likely obtained the drugs illegally. It seems illogical and inconsistent to condemn, even to the point of banning, substances which have proven clinical efficacy in a most intractable condition, simply because non-patients take such drugs in non-therapeutic doses for non-medical reasons. To be consistent, we should similarly ban glue from being used as an adhesive because some misguided teenagers sniff to obtain a particular psychological experience. While I would not for a moment deny that anorectic drugs should be given to obese patients as part of an integrated dietary programme, and then only for patients who are thought to be medically at risk, they can be of real benefit to some of these patients. We are in danger of throwing out the baby of therapeutic efficacy with the bathwater of ill-founded prejudice.

When we come to anorexia nervosa, the clinical features of which are comprehensively reviewed by Szmukler, drugs affecting appetite do not appear to be effective. This is probably because the physiological mechanisms underlying hunger, and consequently the experience of hunger itself, is not usually affected until severe emaciation has occurred. Thus pharmacological manipulation of hunger mechanisms is inappropriate. For this condition, expert and intensive nursing care has been shown to be more effective.

The fact that contributors to this monograph include physiologists, pharmacologists, psychologists, physicians and psychiatrists reflects the complexity of the problem being discussed; namely the ways in which drugs can affect appetite and feeding in human subjects and laboratory animals. This book is presented in the hope that it will help those research workers and clinical practitioners who are wrestling with these matters in their laboratories and/or clinical practices.

Finally I would like to thank all my fellow contributors for making my task as editor so pleasant and rewarding; I for one have certainly learned a great deal.

*October 1981*                                                    T. Silverstone

# ☐ Contents

# 1 □ The Physiology of the Meal

G. P. Smith

Drugs are usually tested for their effects on appetite under restricted conditions. The most common involves adapting a rat to a feeding schedule. When the rat's intake has stabilized on this schedule, then drug treatment begins. The effect of drug treatment is measured by the change in food intake over a short interval (15–120 min usually). A similar paradigm is used with humans except that subjective reports are frequently obtained as well as changes in food intake. Recently, Blundell and his colleagues have begun to measure the effect of drugs on the size and frequency of meals over intervals up to 24 h (see chapter by Blundell and Latham). These paradigms are used to evaluate the acute effect of drugs on meals or short-term food intake. This drug effect is understood in terms of feeding as an episodic behaviour.

Drugs are also administered daily for weeks to determine their effect on body weight. This is the most important therapeutic effect of drugs. This drug effect is understood in terms of feeding as *the* source of nutrient energy for the metabolic arrangements that underlie changes in body weight.

I emphasize the difference between drug effects on meals and on body weight because it is important to grasp that feeding is only one component in the physiological system for body weight. Thus, changes in feeding and changes in body weight are not tightly linked. The tendency for changes in feeding to produce qualitatively similar changes in body weight and the tendency for changes in body weight to produce inverse changes in feeding are most easily observed when large changes occur in feeding or body weight. There is a range of changes in feeding and body weight which metabolic adjustments absorb.

This chapter describes the physiological context in which drugs act on feeding. It deals primarily with the physiology of the most common condition of testing, i.e. the effect of a drug on food intake over an interval of minutes. Since the animal has been adapted to the feeding schedule and the food prior to testing, I shall omit discussion of the physiology of food seeking, food identification, food palatability and conditioning that occurs during the adaption period. The reader should be relieved, there is much to quote and little to say.

## I. THE MEAL

The functional unit of feeding is the meal. The meal is a bout of feeding. Although the termination of a meal is obvious in humans, there has been some debate about a reliable method for deciding that a meal has ended in animals (De Castro, 1975; Kissileff, 1970; Le Magnen and Tallon, 1966; Panksepp, 1976). The discovery of a behavioural sequence that characterizes postprandial satiety (Antin *et al.*, 1975) has resolved the issue, at least under the conditions of animals eating alone in their home cages. When the satiety sequence occurs, the meal has ended.

If we want to understand the physiology of a meal, it is useful to anchor the physiology to feeding behaviour, because the form of the meal is what the physiology must explain. By form of the meal, I mean its beginning, the pattern of ingestion, and its termination. This form is measured directly with ease and precision, particularly with liquid diets.

Because the physiology of a meal is incomplete, I shall also use hypothetical constructs to make the account more coherent. Three constructs are useful for analysing the physiology of a meal. These constructs are the neuropsychological processes of hunger, satiety and reward. Hunger is the process that tends to activate feeding. Satiety is the process that tends to stop feeding. I believe they are complementary processes and that their neural interactions are more complicated than algebraic summation at a single neural site.

Reward is the process that has immediate and delayed effects on feeding. The immediate effect is to sustain feeding. The physiology of this immediate effect is part of the physiology of a meal. The delayed effect is to alter subsequent feeding. The physiology of the delayed effect is not part of the physiology of a meal.

There is nothing original about these constructs. I make them explicit because I refer to them frequently in the rest of this chapter, and it is difficult to know the extent of agreement about them. It is axiomatic that the processes are neuropsychological because the interactions among the psychological phenomena that are decisive for behaviour must involve the central nervous system. The processes are not only neural because the primary experiences of feeding behaviour are psychological, and I believe the psychological is not completely reducible to the neural (see Smith, 1981a for further discussion of these syntactical issues).[a]

---

[a] Given the title of this book, the reader may be curious about my omission of appetite. I omit appetite because appetite usually refers to feeding, in general. Bolles has recently given the historical evidence for this usage (Bolles, 1980). Although some writers assign a more limited meaning to the term in distinguishing hunger and appetite, I have not found the distinction useful. The distinction has not helped the physiological analysis and, as a descendant of the nineteenth century categories of need and want, it has been imposed prematurely on discussions of hunger and other motivations.

## II. PHYSIOLOGY OF THE MEAL

Knowledge of the physiological mechanisms for the control of feeding and of body weight is in an interesting stage of development. We have discarded the neurological and metabolic theories that organized research since the Second World War because we demonstrated that they were not sufficient to explain the facts (the glucostatic hypothesis) or because we learned that they were problems, not explanations (the ventromedial and lateral hypothalamic syndromes, the gastric theory of hunger). This transcendence of previous paradigms coincided with a burst of technical developments in neuroscience and endocrinology that permitted more refined experimental measurements. These technical advances have produced a rich, varied and fragmented literature that apparently defies summary statement. But all of the measurements are not *equally* interesting and relevant. The physiology that is most useful is that which concerns the meal because the meal is the functional unit of feeding behaviour in mammals. Although it is possible to have a physiology of a meal without a physiology of body weight, it is not possible to have a physiology of body weight without a physiology of a meal. The literature bristles with evidence of this.

The physiology of feeding that we have is mainly from the rat. We shall use that for the most part. When the same mechanism has been looked for, it has been found in subhuman primates and in man. The human is certainly more than the rat, but he or she is not less.

### A. Initiation of Feeding

The initiation of feeding (measured by latency to feed) is an orderly and inverse function of hours of food deprivation and percent body weight loss (Bolles, 1975). This orderly relationship reinforces the intuition that feeding is initiated by a metabolic deficit. Mayer proposed that the deficit was a decrease in glucose utilization in the ventromedial hypothalamus (Mayer, 1955). This form of the hypothesis has been rejected (Epstein *et al.*, 1975; Smith, 1976; Smith, 1982b). It is clear, however, that decreased glucose utilization (glucoprivation) produced by insulin hypoglycaemia or by 2-deoxy-D-glucose initiated feeding; this is an example of feeding in response to a metabolic deficit. Since this metabolic deficit has not been demonstrated to occur prior to a spontaneous meal under ordinary laboratory conditions, the glucoprivic mechanism is currently considered an unusual mechanism for initiating feeding that is active only during a metabolic emergency (Smith, 1982b; and see below).

Le Magnen (1980) has an opposing view. He considers a small decrease in blood glucose that occurs regularly just before a spontaneous meal (Louis-Sylvestre and Le Magnen, 1980), to be "definitive evidence for the hypoglycaemia induced glucopenia as a stimulus of the hunger arousal of eating (Le Magnen, 1980, p. 66)". But the size of the decrease is too small to affect glucose utilization, so that this proposal requires a receptor mechanism adequate to detect small changes in *circulating* glucose. The site and function of such a receptor mechanism has not been demonstrated. Furthermore, the proposal ignores the numerous studies in which constant infusions of glucose have maintained blood glucose at high and constant levels and yet these glucose infusions have not prevented the initiation of feeding. There must be some relationship between glucose metabolism and feeding. The point is to make that relationship explicit and physiologically rigorous. Le Magnen's suggestion is explicit, but the evidence for it is not rigorous.

Glucoprivic feeding is the only paradigm in which a metabolic deficit produced by an endogenous hormone elicits the human experience of hunger and the initiation of feeding (Smith, 1982b). For that reason, it continues to be analysed. Recent work on this phenomenon has focussed on the site of receptors, central mechanisms, and the phenomenon of glucoprivic feeding.

There is considerable evidence for peripheral and central receptors (Himsworth, 1970; Niijima, 1969; Novin *et al.*, 1973; Miselis and Epstein, 1975; Rezek *et al.*, 1977; Oomura *et al.*, 1975; Stricker *et al.*, 1977). The central receptors appear to be necessary. Woods and McKay (1978) demonstrated this by using intraventricular injections of alloxan to destroy the central receptors. After alloxan treatment, the feeding response to 2-DG and to insulin hypoglycaemia was markedly reduced or abolished. Such alloxan treatment did not affect daily food intake or body weight. Alloxan-treated rats, however, do eat less after 24 h of food deprivation. These observations are consistent with the view that glucoprivic feeding is a control of feeding during metabolic emergencies, but it is not a control of spontaneous feeding (see above).

The central receptors for the feeding response to central 2-DG have been assumed to be in the hypothalamus (Himsworth, 1970). But Slusser *et al.* (1980), using a glucose analogue, 5-thioglucose, that is more than 10 times as potent as 2-DG for eliciting feeding, found that blockade of the cerebral aqueduct blocked the feeding response to 5-thioglucose administered in the lateral cerebral ventricle, but not the feeding response to subcutaneous 2-DG. This is evidence that the receptors for glucoprivic feeding are in the vicinity of the fourth ventricle.

Analysis of the central mechanisms mediating glucoprivic feeding has revealed two important points: (A) the central mechanisms for feeding in response to 2-DG and to insulin hypoglycaemia can be dissociated by lesions in the zona incerta (Walsh and Grossman, 1975). This demonstrates that the central system mediating the feeding response to these two glucoprivic conditions are not identical. (B) there is convergent evidence that central noradrenergic mechanisms are necessary for glucoprivic feeding.

First, norepinephrine turnover increases during glucoprivation and does not return to normal until feeding occurs (Bellin and Ritter, 1979). Secondly, intraventricular administration of the alpha-adrenergic antagonist phenoxybenzamine blocks glucoprivic feeding (Müller *et al.*, 1972; Berthoud and Mogenson, 1977). Thirdly, injection of norepinephrine (NE) elicits feeding in sated rats through an alpha receptor mechanism in the medial hypothalamus (Leibowitz, 1975; 1978). Fourthly, NE is released from the hypothalamus during its perfusion with 2-DG and insulin (McCaleb *et al.*, 1979).

The third area of promising investigation is the phenomenon of postgluco-privic feeding discovered by Ritter *et al.* (1978). The phenomenon is that rats still eat more when they are not given access to food until 6 to 8 h after the induction of glucoprivation by 2-DG or insulin hypoglycaemia. Ritter *et al.* (1978) call this postglucoprivic feeding because by 6 to 8 h, the blood glucose changes (and presumably cellular glucose utilization) have returned to normal. This postglucoprivic feeding was not abolished by glucose administration that restored blood glucose to normal after hypoglycaemia had occurred, but it was abolished by a bout of feeding during glucoprivation. This phenomenon is interesting as a demonstration of a "metabolic memory" for a glucoprivic deficit that affects feeding. Such a memory process seems necessary for co-ordinating intermittent meals and continuous energy expenditure.

We are left with acute glucoprivation as the only established mechanism for the initiation of feeding. Since this mechanism appears to operate only during metabolic emergencies, we are left without a mechanism for the initiation of any spontaneous meal in any mammal.

The problem is difficult no matter how the initiation of feeding is conceived. If the initiation of feeding is conceived as the response to a metabolic deficit, the problem is to measure the deficit at the critical site. We have no clue about the deficit or the site. If the initiation of feeding is conceived as a response to a psychological process such as learning, memory, anticipation of metabolic deficits (Booth, 1981) or to non-specific arousal (Robbins and Fray, 1980), the problem is to discover an adequate physiological mechanism for these pro-cesses. We haven't a clue here either.

There is one way to conceive the problem that is easier to deal with. That is to conceive the initiation of feeding as primarily determined by the decline of the satiety mechanisms activated by previously ingested food. By definition, these mechanisms tend to inhibit feeding. It is reasonable to assume that their action declines as a function of the time since the meal that activated them. The major evidence for this possibility is that under conditions of *ad libitum* access to food, there is a significant correlation between the amount of food ingested in a meal and the postprandial interval of non-feeding (IMI) that occurs until the initiation of the next meal (Le Magnen and Tallon, 1966). It is clear that the decay of satiety mechanisms is not the only factor that determines when the next meal will begin because the correlation between meal size and post-prandial IMI only accounts for slightly more than half of the variance. But given the lack of clues about how to analyse meal initiation more directly in terms of metabolic deficits or psychological processes, it is worth considering the mechanisms of postprandial satiety as being concerned with both the termination of meals and the initiation of meals. With this possibility in mind, let us consider the physiological mechanisms for postprandial satiety.

## B. Postprandial Satiety

The physiological analysis of the termination of feeding is more accessible than the analysis of the initiation of feeding because we know the adequate stimuli

for the termination of feeding-ingested food provides them. Given that food
provides the adequate stimuli for the termination of feeding, the physiological
analysis depends on the answers to four questions (Table I).

**Table I**.  Questions about the termination of feeding.

(1)  Where do food stimuli act?
(2)  Which food stimuli are adequate?
(3)  What neural and/or endocrine mechanisms are activated?
(4)  What central mechanisms respond to and integrate the peripheral mechanisms?

### (1)  Where Do Food Stimuli Act?

Food stimuli act preabsorptively and postabsorptively to inhibit feeding behaviour. The preabsorptive sites extend from the mouth to the end of the small
intestine. There is evidence for three functionally distinct receptor compart-
ments: pregastric, gastric, and intestinal. Food can act in each of these com-
partments to inhibit feeding. When food acts at more than one compartment,
there is a synergistic action of the individual inhibitory effects. Thus, as ingested
food passes from the mouth down the gut, it activates preabsorptive inhibitory
mechanisms sequentially so that for some time during and after a meal, there is
a period of simultaneous activation of receptor sites. The importance of
sequential activation for optimal inhibition by food can be appreciated best
from the results with preloads. The inhibitory effect of preloading the stomach
(Baile *et al.*, 1971; Quartermain *et al.*, 1971) or intestine (Antin *et al.*, 1977)
with food on subsequent food intake is an inverse function of the duration of
the interval between preload and the initiation of feeding. Short intervals result
in larger inhibitory effects, presumably because they permit more synergism
between inhibitory mechanisms by activating them simultaneously.

  In addition to these preabsorptive sites for the activation of inhibitory
mechanisms, there are postabsorptive sites. There is now strong evidence that
the liver is a postabsorptive site (Booth and Jarman, 1976; Novin and Vanderweele, 1977; Rezek and Novin, 1977). If plausibility were proof, the brain
would also be an important postabsorptive site for the inhibition of feeding by
food stimuli. But the only evidence for the brain as a receptor site is the
presence of hypothalamic receptors sensitive to the iontopheretic application
of glucose and fatty acids (Oomura, 1976). The function of these receptors in
the termination of feeding, however, has never been demonstrated.

### (2)  Which Food Stimuli are Adequate?

Taste, texture, physical chemical, nutrient chemical and mechanical stimuli
have all been demonstrated to inhibit feeding from some preabsorptive or
postabsorptive site (Smith and Gibbs, 1979), but there is very little detailed

knowledge of the relative potency of these stimuli or of their specificity for preabsorptive and postabsorptive receptor sites.

### (3) What Neural and/or Endocrine Mechanisms are Activated?

(a) *Preabsorptive Satiety.* It is best to consider mechanisms by site at which food stimuli act. Activation of pregastric sites alone occurs during sham feeding (Young *et al.*, 1974). Sham feeding activates taste fibres of the facial nerve and afferents of the glossopharyngeal and vagus nerves. Sham feeding also releases hormones such as gastrin and insulin (Fischer *et al.*, 1972). These hormonal responses are blocked by abdominal vagotomy, but the inhibitory effect of sham-fed food on sham feeding is not (Kraly, 1979). This suggests that the neural afferent feedback from above the diaphragm is the major mechanism for terminating a sham-fed meal.

Activation of gastric mechanisms by gastric infusion, by ingestion, or by physical distention produces inhibition of feeding (Smith and Gibbs, 1979). Deutsch *et al.* (1980) have recently suggested that there are distinct gastric mechanisms sensitive to nutrients and to volume. It has been assumed that the vagal afferents from gastric receptors carried the inhibitory signals to the brain, but in the case of ingested liquid food, abdominal vagotomy that spared the hepatic branch did not change the inhibitory effect (Kraly and Gibbs, 1980). This leaves the sympathetic afferents and gastric hormones as possible mediators. The sympathetic afferents have not been evaluated, but the gastric hormones have. Gastrin has no inhibitory effect on feeding (Lorenz *et al.*, 1979), but bombesin does (Gibbs *et al.*, 1979; Martin and Gibbs, 1980). Furthermore, the inhibitory effect of bombesin, like the inhibitory effect of food in the stomach, is not altered by abdominal vagotomy (Gibbs *et al.*, 1980). Thus, bombesin is a putative mechanism for the non-vagal inhibition of feeding by food stimuli in the stomach, but it is far from proven to do this.

Activation of intestinal mechanisms by intestinal infusions inhibits real feeding (Smith and Gibbs, 1979) and sham feeding (Liebling *et al.*, 1975). Despite the evidence for intestinal chemoreceptors of vagal (Mei *et al.*, 1973) and sympathetic afferents (Sharma and Nasset, 1962), the role of neural afferents for "intestinal satiety" (Smith *et al.*, 1974) has not been investigated.

On the other hand, the numerous hormones that are synthesized, stored and released by intestinal mucosal cells (Bloom, 1978) have been extensively tested. Cholecystokinin (CCK) is the only intestinal hormone known to have a potent and reliable inhibitory effect on feeding (Smith, 1980; Smith and Gibbs, 1981). (Bombesin is present in the intestine, but in less quantity than in the stomach.) Secretin and gastric inhibitory polypeptide (gastric insulintropic peptide) have had no effect (Lorenz *et al.*, 1979). The inhibitory effect of CCK (the synthetic octapeptide, CCK-8, has been used extensively) has been demonstrated in a variety of animals (Smith and Gibbs, 1979) and in lean (Kissileff *et al.*, 1981) and fat (Pi-Sunyer *et al.*, 1981) young men.

CCK not only inhibits feeding; CCK elicits the behaviour sequence of satiety in the sham feeding rat (Antin *et al.*, 1975). The doses of CCK that inhibit feeding do not inhibit drinking. The satiety effect requires the same molecular structure that other biological actions of CCK require and it does not appear to be a toxic side effect.

The site of action for the satiety effect is controversial. It appears to be in the abdomen in the rat because abdominal vagotomy markedly reduces or abolishes it (Smith *et al.*, 1979; Smith *et al.*, 1981). On the other hand, Della-Fera and Baile (1979) reported that the infusion of CCK-8 into the cerebro-ventricular system of sheep inhibits feeding, but identical infusions in the rats did not. Della-Fera and Baile (1979) suggest that CCK, synthesized and stored in the brain, is released into the cerebrospinal fluid and acts at some brain site in the sheep to inhibit feeding. The relationship of this interesting effect in sheep to the effect of peripherally administered CCK-8 in other animals and man is not clear at this time. At the very least, it suggests that peripherally administered CCK-8 may exert some of its inhibitory action by a direct effect on the brain, but the failure of ventricular infusions of CCK-8 to inhibit feeding in the rat and the failure of CCK-8 to inhibit feeding after abdominal vagotomy in the rat are serious obstacles for this idea. Only further work can clarify this aspect of the problem.

It is important to emphasize that the evidence for CCK mediating intestinal satiety, at least in part, is all circumstantial. From the effect of abdominal vagotomy on the satiety effect of CCK, however, we already know that CCK is not necessary for the termination of feeding because abdominal vagotomized rats do not overeat. CCK, if it is a satiety signal from the small intestine, is not the only one.

Food stimuli in the small intestine also elicit the release of the pancreatic hormones, insulin and glucagon. This is done through neural and hormonal mechanisms and constitutes the "entero-insular axis" (Pfeiffer *et al.*, 1973). Both immunoreactive insulin and pancreatic glucagon are released during the average meal in the rat so that both are putative satiety signals. Vanderwĕele *et al.* (1980) and Anika *et al.* (1980) have recently reported that exogenous insulin can inhibit food intake. The specificity and mechanisms of the inhibitory effect have not been determined.

The inhibitory effect of glucagon on feeding has been studied since the 1950s. Then it was found that glucagon inhibited gastric contractions and increased arteriovenous (a-v) glucose differences (Stunkard *et al.*, 1955). Within the context of the theories of gastric hunger contractions and of the glucostatic hypothesis, these two effects predicted that glucagon would inhibit food intake in humans. That prediction was fulfilled in two studies in a small number of patients (Penick and Hinkle, 1961; Schulman *et al.*, 1957). In the course of these experiments, however, Penick and Hinkle (1961) noted a temporal dissociation between the inhibitory effect of glucagon on food intake and the increase of a-v glucose difference. This suggested that the inhibitory effect on food intake was not a result of glucagon's effect on glucose metabolism. That question is still open (see below).

A series of animal studies were undertaken simultaneously to analyse the mechanism of glucagon's inhibition of food intake. Repeated injections inhibited food intake and decreased body weight (Salter, 1960). Part of the weight loss during repeated glucagon injections is probably due to the increased metabolic rate that glucagon produces (Davidson *et al.*, 1960). Novin and his colleagues revived interest in this effect of glucagon. They showed that single injections of glucagon inhibited food intake, but did not inhibit food-related drinking. Furthermore, glucagon did not serve as an unconditioned stimulus for a conditioned taste aversion (Martin and Novin, 1977).

The most common mechanism proposed for glucagon's inhibitory effect is hepatic glycogenolysis. The major evidence for this is the observation that the inhibitory effect of glucagon is diminished or abolished by overnight deprivation periods (Vanderweele *et al.*, 1979) and that such deprivations reduce hepatic glycogen. Since abdominal vagotomy blocks the inhibitory effect of glucagon (Martin *et al.*, 1978; Vanderweele *et al.*, 1979), it has been suggested that some metabolic event associated with hepatic glycogenolysis is detected by vagal afferent nerves in the liver and relayed to the brain (Novin and Vanderweele, 1977; Russek, 1971). Geary *et al.* (1980) provided indirect support for glucose metabolic changes being critical for the inhibitory effect of glucagon by demonstrating that glucagon's effects on lipid metabolism are not necessary for its inhibitory effect on food intake.

(b) *Postabsorptive Satiety*. There is evidence that the liver is a site where absorbed carbohydrate produces an inhibitory effect on feeding through a vagal afferent mechanism (Novin and Vanderweele, 1977). It has been occasionally suggested that amino acids and fats inhibit feeding, but there is no evidence for such effects in postprandial satiety.

The possibility exists that glucose or other circulating nutrients act directly on the brain to inhibit feeding. Oomura (1976) has demonstrated hypothalamic units that apparently have the required sensitivity and specificity. But no one has demonstrated a relationship between the activity of such units and postprandial satiety.

(c) *Gastric Emptying and the Co-ordination of Peripheral Satiety Mechanisms*. Having considered the neural and hormonal mechanisms that *might* mediate the satiety effect of food stimuli, let us consider how gastric emptying co-ordinates them. This co-ordinating function of gastric emptying derives from the fact that gastric emptying is the rate-limiting function for the distribution of ingested food between the stomach and the small intestine. Since the capacity of the small intestine to absorb nutrients is larger than the usual rate of delivery of nutrients by gastric emptying, the rate of delivery of nutrients to postabsorptive sites also depends on the rate of gastric emptying (Johansson, 1975). Schusdziarra *et al.* (1980) recently reported that the gut hormone somatostatin could change the rate of absorption. This is the only known mechanism that could intervene between emptying and absorption.

Given its pivotal position, it is attractive to relate the control of gastric emptying (Cooke, 1975) to the control of food intake. Since gastric emptying is increased by the volume of ingested food, feeding controls emptying. But, when emptying slows as the result of neuroendocrine feedback from food stimuli that emptied into the small intestine, it is possible that the decreased emptying decreases food intake. This has been viewed for a long time as a mechanical effect. Decreased emptying during feeding produces increased gastric distention; this activates vagal afferents, and the central effect of such vagal afferent activity is to inhibit feeding (Paintal, 1973; Towbin, 1955). We have discussed the recent report of Kraly and Gibbs (1980) that contradicts this proposal.

An alternative possibility is that distention produced by decreased gastric emptying inhibits feeding through hormonal mechanisms. The hormonal mechanisms could be those from the intestine that inhibit gastric emptying (e.g. CCK, secretin, GIP) or those from the stomach that are released by distention (gastrin, VIP and, possibly bombesin). Two of these hormones, CCK and bombesin, inhibit food intake but VIP apparently does not (Gibbs, personal communication). McHugh and Moran have emphasized the role of gastric emptying in the control of food intake, and they have suggested that the satiety effect of CCK depends upon its inhibition of gastric emptying (McHugh, 1979; Moran and McHugh, 1979). The fact that abdominal vagotomy blocks both effects of CCK (Smith *et al.*, 1979; Yamagishi and Debas, 1978) supports their suggestion; the ability of CCK to inhibit sham feeding (Gibbs *et al.*, 1973), a situation in which gastric emptying into the intestine is prevented by draining food out of the stomach, is not consistent with the satiety effect being dependent on gastric emptying. The question is open and important. New experiments are required to determine if the inhibitory effects of intestinal hormones on feeding and on gastric emptying are parallel effects or sequential effects.

## (4) *What Central Mechanisms Respond to and Integrate the Peripheral Mechanisms?*

*Central Mechanisms of Postprandial Satiety.* Until the last 5 years, it had been widely accepted that the ventromedial hypothalamus (VMH) was an important central site for satiety. The evidence for this was the dramatic hyperphagia produced by bilateral lesions of the VMH (Hetherington and Ranson, 1940) and the claim by Miller *et al.* (1950) that VMH hyperphagia rats had a specific deficit in satiety without a change in hunger. This influential inference was based on the observation that VMH rats ate more than normal when little effort was required to obtain food, but they ate less than normal when access to food required a large number of responses. But when VMH rats are adapted to the operant situation and their food intake is restricted so that they are tested in the dynamic phase of hyperphagia, VMH rats show decreased latency to feed (Sclafani, 1972) and increased intake even when the operant requirements are difficult (Sclafani and Kluge, 1974). This suggests that they *are* more hungry. Furthermore, when the peripheral satiety mechanisms are stimulated by preloads, VMH rats or monkeys respond normally (Thomas and Mayer, 1968; McHugh *et al.*, 1975; Panksepp, 1971). These and other data have led to open scepticism about the satiety function of the VMH. A new view of the syndrome that emphasizes peripheral neuroendrocrine and visceral changes is now current (Powlcy, 1977). The major advantage to the new view is that the VMH syndrome is now seen as a problem to be solved instead of an explanation to be invoked. The problem is twofold. First, we must account for the hyperphagia neuropsychologically. Hyperphagia could be the result of increased hunger, decreased satiety, and/or increased reward. Secondly, we must account for the hyperphagia physiologically. Our inability to explain VMH hyperphagia is a consequence of our inadequate understanding of the physiology of a normal meal. Without the normal physiology, it is not easy to know what is disturbed by the VMH lesions. Our ignorance is extensive, and fundamental.

Monoamine neurons may form part of the central satiety mechanisms. There is considerable evidence that activation of central serotonin mechanisms inhibits feeding (see chapters by Blundell and Latham, and by Samanin and Garattini). The catecholamines may also be involved at the hypothalamic level. Ahlskog and Hoebel (1973) demonstrated hyperphagia after lesion of the ventral noradrenergic bundle. Leibowitz and Rossakis (1978, 1979) inhibited feeding by dopamine (DA) and epinephrine injections into perifornical hypothalamic sites. Leibowitz considers the release of DA at perifornical sites to be critical for the anorexic effect of amphetamine. However, oral administration of the DA receptor-blocking drug pimozide failed to reduce the anorectic effect of small doses of dextroamphetamine in man (see chapter by Silverstone and Kyriakides).

The observation of increased release of NE (McCaleb et al., 1979) and DA (Martin and Myers, 1976; Heffner et al., 1980) from hypothalamic sites during feeding is consistent with the postulated role in satiety. The increased release of DA in the amygdala reported by Heffner et al. (1980) after gastric loads of saline or food may also be relevant to central satiety mechanisms.

I hope it is clear that none of these monaminergic systems has been linked to satiety unambiguously. Inhibition of feeding may not only be due to increased satiety; it may also be due to decreased hunger and/or decreased reward. None of the experiments has distinguished among these possibilities.

## C. Food Reward

The immediate reward value of food that affects meal size is usually discussed in terms of preferred taste stimuli or, more broadly, palatability. From the standpoint of physiological control, it is food-contingent positive feedback. Wiepkema (1971) has demonstrated this phenomenon in the early part of a meal in mice.

Given the fundamental importance of the pleasures of feeding and its reward value in behaviour and psychological theory, it is surprising that the physiological analysis of this aspect of food-contingent stimuli has not received much experimental attention. The analysis of food as a reward has been mostly behavioural and psychological. It has been carried out primarily by investigating the effect of changes in the quantity and taste of food, and the pattern of responses required for access to it on the acquisition, performance and/or extinction of those responses (Collier, 1962; Collier and Siskel, 1959; Collier and Myers, 1961; Weiskrantz and Cowey, 1963; Weiskrantz and Baltzer, 1963). But since immediate reward is apparently food-contingent, the physiological analysis of reward could be guided by the same questions that provided the structure for our analysis of satiety as a food contingent process (see Section II B). Taking this approach emphasizes the possible relationships between satiety and reward. Taking this approach also opens up for investigation the peripheral and central physiological distinctions between the neuropsychological processes of satiety and reward.

The mouth and the stomach are the only two gut sites that have been demonstrated to be involved in food reward. Preferred tastes have immediate reward and can sustain feeding when satiety mechanisms are experimentally minimized. The most vivid example of this is the 17 h deprived rat that sham feeds almost continuously for hours (Young et al., 1974). Miller and Kessen (1952) showed that food intubated into the stomach could serve as a reward. The reward value of intragastric food was less than orally ingested food. Holman (1968) opposed the stomach as a site of reward and claimed that the reward value of intragastric food was a result of the enhancement of oral food reward.

It is not possible to decide this question at this time, but the recent work of Puerto et al. (1976) is relevant. They demonstrated that intragastric injections of milk mixed with gastric secretions had a reward effect, but isovolumetric injections of whole milk, glucose or saline did not. Deutsch and Wang (1977) extended this work by showing that when food in the stomach was prevented from entering the small intestine by an inflated cuff around the pylorus, food still produced reward. This, I believe, is all we know about the sites of food reward. There is nothing known about the nature of the adequate stimuli except for the sweet taste of foods. And, except for the neuroanatomy and neurophysiology of the peripheral taste system, nothing is known about the peripheral neural and/or endocrine mechanisms that mediate food reward.

In addition to the central pathways for taste (Norgren and Leonard, 1973), the central dopaminergic system has been recently suggested as a central mechanism for food reward by Wise et al. (1978). Their major evidence is that omitting the food reward or pretreatment with the dopamine antagonist pimozide produces very similar effects on performance of a food-reinforced operant. Although prior reports of such an effect had been interpreted as a motor deficit, I believe the results of Wise et al. (1978) make the motor deficit interpretation unlikely. If the hypothesis of Wise is correct, then central DA neurons must be active during feeding. Martin and Myers (1976) found evidence of DA release in the hypothalamus during feeding, but Vander-Gugten et al. (1977) did not. Biggio et al. (1977) measured brain changes in two DA metabolites (3, 4 dihydroxyphenylacetic acid, DOPAC; and homovanillic acid, HVA) and found that they increased during a 3-h feeding period and remained elevated for several hours after feeding ended. Since the changes in these metabolites, particularly DOPAC, reflect changes in DA neuronal activity

(Roth *et al.*, 1976), these results are evidence that central DA neurons are more active during and after feeding than they are during the period of food deprivation that precedes feeding.

Heffner *et al.* (1980) have recently made a clear demonstration of the increase in central DA neuronal activity during feeding. Using the ratio of the concentration of DOPAC to the concentration of DA as an index of DA neuronal activity, they found that 1 h of feeding in which about 20 g of food was consumed was correlated with significant increases in the DOPAC/DA ratio in n. accumbens, posterior hypothalamus and amygdala, but *not* in other DA terminal fields such as the striatum, frontal cortex, olfactory tubercle or septum. When food or saline was intubated into the stomach, the results were even more specific: the DOPAC/DA ratio increased only in the amygdala.

Heffner *et al.* (1980) emphasized that they did not know what food stimuli produced these changes and they did not know what food contingent process (satiety, reward, motor performance) the changes in dopaminergic activity were mediating. Their caution is appropriate, but the work is at least consistent with central DA mechanisms mediating food reward.

## III. PHYSIOLOGY OF BODY WEIGHT

Now we move from the meal to the scale. The control of body weight is known to involve more factors and operate over a longer span of time than the control of feeding. The metabolic disposition of ingested food complicates the relationship between the meal and the scale. It is the capacity of nutrient metabolism to vary that permits feeding behaviour and meal patterns to adapt to such varied demands for the energy in food as lactation, growth, changes in environmental temperature, and changes in the availability of food. For feeding to serve energy exchange, the controls of feeding must be embedded in the neuroendocrine controls of metabolism. Logic and intuition carry the problem this far. But logic and intuition do not help to identify the mechanisms or to explicate the hierarchy of control. The plausible linkages between the physiology of meals and of body weight include the neuroendocrine controls of metabolism (e.g., insulin, glucagon, and growth hormone), the rate of metabolism (glucose utilization, ATP utilization), the storage of nutrient (fat), the rate of delivery of nutrient for metabolic disposition (gastric emptying) and/or metabolic products (lactic acid). Since none of these has been demonstrated rigorously and none of them has been excluded, it is beyond the scope of this chapter to review the evidence for the relative importance of any of these metabolic mechanisms.

I want to emphasize a neglected aspect of this problem that is an obvious deduction from the fact that feeding behaviour serves metabolism and nutrition. That is that whatever metabolic controls act on feeding, they must have access to the mechanisms that control meals. This very obvious point has received little experimental attention. This failure to attempt to explain disorders of the control of meals prevents our literature from reflecting the important linkage between meals and the scale.

The beginnings of such explanations can be seen in the meal patterns of rodents that have hyperphagic obesity on a genetic basis or on the basis of ventromedial hypothalamic (VMH) lesions or VMH disconnections. All of these hyperphagic obese rodents eat larger meals and, to a lesser extent, eat more frequently. It should now be possible to begin to determine what changes in which neuropsychological processes (hunger, satiety or reward) underlie the changes in meal patterns. The investigation of the relative increased feeding at night in the rat by Kraly *et al.* (1980) is an example of what might be learned from such an approach. They found no evidence that rats were hungrier at night, but they found clear evidence that peripheral satiety signals were less potent at night. Whether the decreased potency of satiety signals is a result of *decreased* sensitivity of the central satiety system and/or an *increased* sensitivity of the reward system remains to be determined. This work is cited primarily to indicate the heuristic value of such an approach to hyperphagic obesity and other disorders of body weight.

## IV. PHYSIOLOGY OF FEEDING AND DRUG ACTION

Realization that the termination of feeding is dependent upon stimuli of ingested food contacting preabsorptive and postabsorptive sites provides a new view for thinking about anorectic agents. For example, it should be possible to develop anorectics that act at preabsorptive sites and are never absorbed. Secondly, even if the anorectic had to be absorbed to become active, it would not need to act directly on the brain. Both of these characteristics would enhance specificity and safety. The preabsorptive mechanisms have the requisite specificity; a number of the manipulations that inhibit feeding have no effect on drinking. This is even true when the food is in liquid form so that the motor acts of ingestion are apparently identical for feeding and drinking (Smith and Gibbs, 1981).

Gut hormones could be exploited as anorectic agents in two ways. First, endogenous hormones could be released by calorically trivial amounts of a specific stimulus ingested just before a meal. This would result in a synergistic interaction between the hormone released and the satiety mechanisms activated by ingested food. This synergistic interaction should terminate a meal sooner; thus, less food would be eaten. This strategy has been tested by giving L-phenylalanine, a strong stimulant of CCK release, to monkeys (Gibbs *et al.*, 1976) and to humans (Fincham *et al.*, 1977). The monkeys ate significantly less and the humans felt significantly less hungry. The result in monkeys was controlled by giving equal loads of D-phenylalanine. D-phenylalanine is a weak stimulant of CCK release; D-phenylalanine did not inhibit feeding.

The second way to exploit gut hormones as anorectic agents is to administer them just before a meal. An example of this strategy is the inhibition of meal size produced by intravenous infusions of CCK-8 in lean and obese humans (Kissileff *et al.*, 1981, Pi-Sunyer *et al.*, 1981).

The realization of the prominence of peripheral mechanisms for satiety increases the possible explanations for the anorectic effect of drugs that affect brain monoamine systems (Samanin and Garattini's chapter). For example, an anorectic could affect the peripheral mechanisms directly by an effect on monoamine systems in the gut. Or an anorectic could affect the peripheral mechanisms indirectly through an effect on the central monoamine mechanisms that are activated by the peripheral mechanisms. Anorectic agents could also affect the peripheral mechanisms through the visceral effects that are produced by a change in central monoamine mechanisms. Any of these effects of monoamine manipulation may be involved in the differential inhibition of food stimuli that underlies nutrient selection (see Blundell and Latham).

Finally, I believe the problem of predicting the effectiveness of an anorectic agent for reducing body weight from its ability to decrease meal size is related to our current failure to articulate the physiology of meals with the physiology of body weight. Until a common physiology is achieved, the evaluation of anorectics will remain starkly empiric. There are two reasons for this: first, we don't know what meal control mechanisms have been affected by an anorectic drug. Secondly, we don't know how the sensitivity of these mechanisms to the anorectic drug will be altered by the metabolic changes associated with loss of weight during a therapeutic trial.

On the other hand, anorectic drugs can serve an analytic purpose because drugs are chemically specified, cellular probes of the physiological control systems. By tracking their effectiveness on specific controls of feeding across a range of metabolic situations, anorectic drugs will chip away our fundamental ignorance. The chapters that follow contain numerous examples of relationships between drugs and their effects on the meal and the scale.

## ACKNOWLEDGEMENTS

I thank my colleagues at the Bourne Laboratory for their criticisms of this manuscript and Ms Nina DiFilippo and Mrs Ellen Andrews for typing the manuscript. I wrote this during the tenure of Research Scientist Development Award MH 00149.

## REFERENCES

Ahlskog, J. E. and Hoebel, B. G. (1973). Overeating and obesity from damage to a noradrenergic system in the brain. *Science* **182**, 166–169.

Anika, S. M., Houpt, T. R. and Houpt, K. A. (1980). Insulin as a satiety hormone. *Physiol. Behav.* **25**, 21–23.

Antin, J., Gibbs, J., Holt, J., Young, R. C. and Smith, G. P. (1975). Cholecystokinin elicits the complete behavioral sequence of satiety in rats. *J. Comp. Physiol. Psychol.* **89**, 784–790.

Antin, J., Gibbs, J. and Smith, G. P. (1977). Intestinal satiety requires pregastric food stimulation. *Physiol. Behav.* **18**, 421–425.

Baile, C. A., Zinn, W. and Mayer, J. (1971). Feeding behavior of monkeys: glucose utilization rate and site of glucose entry. *Physiol. Behav.* **6**, 537–541.

Bellin, S. I. and Ritter, S. (1979). Insulin-induced elevation of hypothalamic NE turnover persists after glucorestoration unless feeding occurs. *Soc. for Neuroscience Abstracts* **5**, 213.

Berthoud, H. R. and Mogenson, G. J. (1977). Ingestive behaviour after intracerebral and intracerebraventricular infusions of glucose and 2-deoxy-D-glucose. *Am. J. Physiol.* **233**, R127–R133.

Biggio, G., Porcedder, M. L., Fratta, W. and Gessa, G. L. (1977). Changes in dopamine metabolism associated with fasting and satiation. *Adv. Biochem. Psycholpharm.* **16**, 377–383.

Bloom, S. R. (ed.), (1978). *In* "Gut Hormones". Churchill Livingstone, Edinburgh, London and New York.

Bolles, R. C. (1975). *In* "Theory of Motivation". Harper & Row, New York.

Bolles, R. C. (1980). Historical note on the term "appetite". *Appetite*, **1**, 3–6.

Booth, D. A. and Jarman, S. P. (1976). Inhibition of food intake in the rat following complete absorption of glucose delivered into the stomach, intestine or liver. *J. Physiol.* (London) **259**, 501–522.

Booth, D. A. (1981). Hunger and satiety as conditioned reflexes. *In* "Brain, Behavior and Bodily Disease". (H. Weiner, M. A. Hofer and A. J. Stunkard, eds), pp. 143–163. Raven Press, New York.

Collier, G. (1962). Some properties of saccharin as a reinforcer. *J. exp. Psychol.* **64**, 184–191.

Collier, G. and Myers, L. (1961). The loci of reinforcement. *J. exp. Psychol.* **61**, 57–66.

Collier, G. and Siskel, Jr, M. (1959). Performance as a joint function of amount of reinforcement and inter-reinforcement interval. *J. exp. Psychol.* **57**, 115–120.

Cooke, A. R. (1975). Control of gastric emptying and motility. *Gastroenterology* **68**, 804–816.

Davidson, I. W. F., Salter, J. M. and Best, C. H. (1960). The effect of glucagon on metabolic rate of rats. *Am. J. Clin. Nutr.* **8**, 540–545.

De Castro, J. M. (1975). Meal pattern correlations: Facts and artifacts. *Physiol. Behav.* **15**, 13–15.

Della-Fera, M. A. and Baile, C. A. (1979). Cholecystokinin octapeptide: continuous picomole injections into the cerebral ventricles of sheep suppress feeding. *Science* **206**, 471–473.

Deutsch, J. A. and Wang, M. L. (1977). The stomach as a site for rapid nutrient reinforcement sensors. *Science* **195**, 89–90.

Deutsch, J. A., Gonzalez, M. F. and Young, W. G. (1980). Two factors control meal size. *Brain Res. Bull.* **5**, Suppl, 4, 55–57.

Epstein, A. N., Nicolaidis, S. and Miselis, R. (1975). The glucoprivic control of food intake and the glucostatic theory of feeding behavior. *In* "Neural Integration of Physiological Mechanisms and Behavior" (G. J. Mogenson and F. R. Calaresu, eds), pp. 148–168, University of Toronto Press, Toronto.

Fincham, J., Silverstone, T. and Saha, B. (1977). The effect of L-phenylalanine on subjective hunger and satiety in man. Program, 6th International Conference on the Physiology of Food and Fluid Intake.

Fischer, U., Hommel, H., Ziegler, M. and Jutzi, E. (1972). The mechanism of insulin secretion after oral glucose administration. III. Investigations of the mechanism of a reflectoric insulin mobilization after oral stimulation. *Diabetologia* **8**, 385–390.

Geary, N., Langhaus, W. and Scharrer, E. (1980). Glucagon induced suppression of food intake is associated with hepatic glycogenolysis without lipolysis or ketogenesis. *Soc. for Neuroscience Abstracts* **6**, 517.

Gibbs, J., Falasco, J. D. and McHugh, P. R. (1976). Cholecstokinin-decreased food intake in rhesus monkeys. *Am. J. Physiol.* **230**, 15–18.

Gibbs, J., Fauser, D. J., Rowe, E. A., Rolls, B. J., Rolls, E. T. and Maddison, S. P. (1979). Bombesin suppresses feeding in rats. *Nature* **282**, 208–210.

Gibbs, J., Jerome, C. and Smith, G. P. (1980). Differential effects of vagotomy on bombesin and cholecystokinin-induced satiety. Seventh International Food and Fluid Intake Conference, Warsaw.

Gibbs, J., Young, R. C. and Smith, G. P. (1973). Cholecystokinin elicits satiety in rats with open gastric fistulas. *Nature* (London) **245**, 323–325.

Heffner, T. G., Hartman, J. A. and Seiden, L. S. (1980). Feeding increases dopamine metabolism in the rat brain. *Science* **208**, 1168–1170.

Hetherington, A. W. and Ranson, S. W. (1940). Hypothalamic lesions and adiposity in the rat. *Anat. Rec.* **78**, 149.

Himsworth, R. L. (1970). Hypothalamic control of adrenaline secretion in response to insufficient glucose. *J. Physiol.* (London) **206**, 411–417.

Holman, G. L. (1968). Intragastric reinforcement effect. *J. Comp. Physiol. Psychol.* **69**, 432–441.

Johansson, C. (1975). Studies of gastrointestinal interactions VII. Characteristics of the absorption pattern of sugar, fat and protein from composite meals in man. A quantitative study. *Scand. J. Gastroent.* **10**, 33–42.

Kissileff, H. (1970). Free feeding in normal and recovered lateral rats monitored by a pellet-detecting eatometer. *Physiol. Behav.* **5**, 163–173.

Kissileff, H. R., Pi-Sunyer, F. X., Thornton, J. and Smith, G. P. (1981). Cholecystokinin-octapeptide (CCK-8) decreases food intake in man. *Am. J. Clin. Nutr.* **34**,154–160.

Kraly, F. S. (1979). Abdominal vagotomy disrupts drinking elicited by pregastric food-contingent stimulation in rats. *Soc. for Neuroscience Abstracts* **5**, 219.

Kraly, F. S. and Gibbs, J. (1980). Vagotomy fails to block the satiating effect of food in the stomach. *Physiol. Behav.* **24**, 1007–1010.

Kraly, F. S., Cushin, B. J. and Smith, G. P. (1980). Nocturnal hyperphagia in the rat is characterized by decreased postprandial satiety. *J. Comp. Physiol. Psychol.* **94**, 375–387.

Leibowitz, S. F. (1975). Ingestion in the satiated rat: role of alpha and beta receptors in mediating effects of hypothalamic adrenergic stimulation. *Physiol. Behav.* **14**, 743–754.

Leibowitz, S. F. (1978). Paraventricular nucleus: A primary site mediating adrenergic stimulation of feeding and drinking. *Pharmacol. Biochem. Behav.* **8**, 163–175.

Leibowitz, S. F. and Rossakais, C. (1978). Pharmacological characterization of perifornical hypothalamic $\beta$-adrenergic receptors mediating feeding inhibition in the rat. *Neuropharmacol.* **17**, 691–702.

Leibowitz, S. F. and Rossakis, C. (1979). Mapping study of brain dopamine- and epinephrine-sensitive sites which cause feeding suppression in the rat. *Brain Res.* **172**, 101–113.

Le Magnen, J. (1980). The body energy regulation: The role of three brain responses to glucopenia. *Neurosci. Biobehav. Rev.* **4**, Suppl. 1, 65–72.

Le Magnen, J. and Tallon, S. (1966). La périodicité spontannée de la prise d'aliments ad libitum du rat blanc. *J. Physiol.* (Paris) **58**, 323–349.

Liebling, D. S., Eisner, J. D., Gibbs, J. and Smith, G. P. (1975). Intestinal satiety in rats. *J. Comp. Physiol. Psychol.* **89**, 955–965.

Lorenz, D. N., Kreielsheimer, G. and Smith, G. P. (1979). Effect of cholecystokinin, gastrin, secretin and GIP on sham feeding in the rat. *Physiol. Behav.* **23**, 1065–1072.

Louis-Sylvestre, J. and Le Magnen, J. (1980). A fall in blood glucose levels precedes meal onset in free feeding rats. *Neurosci. Biobehav Rev.* **4**, Suppl. 1, 13–15.

Martin, C. F. and Gibbs, J. (1980). Bombesin elicits satiety in sham feeding rats. *Peptides* **1**, 131–134.

Martin, G. E. and Myers, R. D. (1976). Dopamine efflux from the brain stem of the rat during feeding, drinking and lever-pressing for food. *Pharmacol. Biochem. Behav.* **4**, 551–560.

Martin, J. R. and Novin, D. (1977). Decreased feeding in rats following hepatic-portal infusion of glucagon. *Physiol. Behav.* **19**, 461–466.

Martin, J. R., Novin, D. and Vanderweele, D. A. (1978). Loss of glucagon suppression of feeding after vagotomy in rats. *Am. J. Physiol.* **234**, E314–E318.

Mayer, J. (1955). Regulation of energy intake and the body weight: The glucostatic theory and the lipostatic hypothesis. *Ann. N.Y. Acad. Sci.* **63**, 15–43.

McCaleb, M. L., Myers, R. D., Singer, G. and Willis, G. (1979). Hypothalamic norepinephrine in the rat during feeding and push-pull perfusion with glucose, 2-DG or insulin. *Am. J. Physiol.* **236**, R312–R321.

McHugh, P. R. (1979). Aspects of the control of feeding: application of quantitation in psychobiology. *Johns Hopkins Med. J.* **144**, 147–155.

McHugh, P. R., Gibbs, J., Falasco, J. D., Moran, T. and Smith, G. P. (1975). Inhibitions on feeding examined in rhesus monkeys with hypothalamic disconnexions. *Brain* **98**, 441–454.

Mei, N., Boyer, A. and Arlhac, A. (1973). Activité unitaire des glucido-récepteurs vagaux de l'intestine. Relation avec la glycémie. *J. de Physiol.* (Paris) **67**, 294A.

Miller, N. E., Bailey, C. J. and Stevenson, J. A. F. (1950). Decreased "hunger" but increased food intake resulting from hypothalamic lesions. *Science* **112**, 256–259.

Miller, N. E. and Kessen, M. L. (1952). Reward effects of food via stomach fistula compared with those of food via mouth. *J. Comp. Physiol. Psychol.* **45**, 555–564.

Miselis, R. and Epstein, A. N. (1975). Feeding induced by intracerebro-ventricular 2-deoxy-D-glucose in the rat. *Am. J. Physiol.* **229**, 1438–1447.

Moran, T. H. and McHugh, P. R. (1980). The dynamics of O-CCK in gastric emptying and feeding. *Program of Eastern Psychol. Assoc.* p. 149.

Müller, E. E., Cocchi, D. and Mantegazza, P. (1972). Brain adrenergic system in the feeding response induced by 2-deoxy-D-glucose. *Am. J. Physiol.* **223**, 945–950.

Niijima, A. (1969). Afferent impulse discharges from glucoreceptors in the guinea pig. *Ann. N.Y. Acad. Sci.* **157**, 690–700.

Norgren, R. and Leonard, C. M. (1973). Ascending central gustatory pathways. *J. Comp. Neur.* **150**, 217–238.

Novin, D. and Vanderweele, D. A. (1977). Visceral involvement in feeding: There is more to regulation than the hypothalamus. *In* "Progress in Psychobiology and Physiological Psychology" (J. M. Sprague and A. N. Epstein, eds ), **7**, 193–241. Academic Press, New York and London.

Novin, D., Vanderweele, D. A. and Rezek, M. (1973). Infusions of 2-deoxy-D-glucose into the hepatic-portal system causes eating: Evidence for peripheral glucoreceptors. *Science* **181**, 858–860.

Oomura, Y., Sugimori, M., Nakamura, T. and Yamada, Y. (1975). Contribution of electrophysiological techniques to the understanding of central control systems. *In* "Neural Integration of Physiological Mechanisms and Behavior" (G. J. Mogenson and F. R. Calaresu, eds), pp. 375–395, University of Toronto Press, Toronto.

Oomura, Y. (1976). Effects of glucose and free fatty acid on the hypothalamic feeding and satiety neurons. *In* "Hunger: Basic Mechanisms and Clinical Implications" (D. Novin, W. Wyrwicka and G. Bray, eds), pp. 145–157, Raven Press, New York.

Paintal, A. S. (1973). Vagal sensory receptors and their reflex effect. *Physiol. Rev.* 53, 159-227.

Panksepp, J. (1971). Is satiety mediated by the ventromedial hypothalamus? *Physiol. Behav.* 7, 381–384.

Panksepp, J. (1976). On the nature of feeding patterns—primarily in rats. *In* "Hunger: Basic Mechanisms and Clinical Implications" (D. Novin, W. Wyrwicka and G. Bray, eds), pp. 369–382, Raven Press, New York.

Penick, S. B. and Hinkle, Jr, L. E. (1961). Depression of food intake induced in healthy subjects by glucagon. *New Eng. J. Med.* 264, 893–897.

Pfeiffer, E. F., Raptis, S. and Fussgänger, R. (1973). Gastrointestinal hormones and islet function. *In* Secretin, Cholecystokinin, Pancreozymin and Gastrin" (J. E. Jorpes and V. Mutt, eds), pp. 259–310, Springer-Verlag, New York.

Pi-Sunyer, F. X., Kissileff, H. R., Thornton, J. and Smith, G. P. (1981). Cholecysto-kinin-octapeptide (CCK-8) decreases food intake in obese men. *Clin. Res.* 29, A631. press).

Powley, T. L. (1977). The ventromedial hypothalamic syndrome, satiety and a cephalic phase hypothesis. *Psychol. Rev.* 84, 89–126.

Puerto, A., Deutsch, J. A., Molina, F. and Roll, P. (1976). Rapid rewarding effects of intragastric injections. *Behav. Biol.* 18, 123–134.

Quartermain, D., Kissileff, H., Shapiro, R. and Miller, N. E. (1971). Suppression of food intake with intragastric loading: relation to natural feeding cycle. *Science* 173, 941–943.

Rezek, M., Kroeger, E. A., Lesnik, H., Havlicek, V. and Novin, D. (1977). Cerebral and hepatic glucoreceptors: assessment of their role in food intake control by the uptake of $^3$H-2-deoxy-D-glucose. *Physiol. Behav.* 18, 679–683.

Rezek, M. and Novin, D. (1977). Hepatic-portal nutrient infusion: effect on feeding in intact and vagotomized rabbits. *Am. J. Physiol.* 232, E119–E130.

Ritter, R. C., Roelke, M. and Neville, M. (1978). Glucoprivic feeding behavior in absence of other signs of glucoprivation. *Am. J. Physiol.* 234, E617–E621.

Robbins, T. W. and Fray, P. J. (1980). Stress-induced eating: fact, fiction or misunder-standing? *Appetite* 1, 103–133.

Roth, R. H., Murrin, L. C. and Walters, J. R. (1976). Central dopaminergic neurons: effects of alterations in impulse flow on the accumulation of dihydroxyphenylacetic acid. *Eur. J. Pharmacol.* 36, 163–171.

Russek, M. (1971). Hepatic receptors and the neurophysiological mechanisms control-ling feeding behavior. *In* "Neurosciences Research" (S. Ehrenpreis and O. C. Solnitzky, eds), 4, 214–282. Academic Press, New York and London.

Salter, J. M. (1960). Metabolic effects of glucagon in the Wistar rat. *Am. J. Clin. Nutr.* 8, 535–539.

Schulman, J. L., Carleton, J. L., Whitney, G. and Whitehorn, J. C. (1957). Effect of glucagon on food intake and body weight in man. *J. Appl. Physiol.* 11, 419–421.

Schusdziarra, V., Zyznar, E., Rouiller, D., Boden, G., Brown, J.C., Arimura, A. and Unger, R. H. (1980). Splanchnic somatostatin: a hormonal regulator of nutrient homeostasis. *Science* 207, 530–532.

Sclafani, A. (1972). The effects of food deprivation and palatability on the latency to eat of normal and hyperphagic rats. *Physiol. Behav.* 8, 977–979.

Sclafani, A. and Kluge, L. (1974). Food motivation and body weight levels in hypo-thalamic hyperphagic rats: a dual lipostat model of hunger and appetite. *J. Comp Physiol. Psyschol.* 86, 28–46.

Sharma, K. N. and Nasset, E. S. (1962). Electrical activity in mesenteric nerves after perfusion of gut lumen. *Am. J. Physiol.* 202, 725–730.

Slusser, P. G., Stone, S. L. and Ritter, R. C. (1980). Glucoreceptors for feeding and hyperglycemia: evidence against their location in the forebrain. *Soc. for Neuroscience* **6**, 127.

Smith, G. P. (1976). Humoral hypotheses for the control of food intake. *In* "Obesity in Perspective" Vol. 2, Part 2, (G. Bray, ed.) pp. 19–29. National Institute of Health, Bethesda, Maryland.

Smith, G. P. (1980). The satiety effect of gastrointestinal hormones. *In* "Polypeptide Hormones" (R. F. Beers, Jr and E. G. Bassett, eds), pp. 413–420. Raven Press, New York.

Smith, G. P. (1982a). Satiety and the problem of motivation. *In* "The Physiological Mechanisms of Motivation" (D. W. Pfaff, ed.), (in press). Springer Verlag, New York.

Smith, G. P. (1982b). Gut hormones and feeding behavior: intuitions and experiments. *In* "Behavioral Neuroendocrinology" (C. Nemeroff and A. Dunn, eds), (in press). Spectrum, Holliswood.

Smith, G. P. and Gibbs, J. (1979). Postprandial satiety. *In* "Progress in Psychobiology and Physiological Psychology" (J. M. Sprague and A. N. Epstein, eds), 179–242. Academic Press, New York and London.

Smith, G. P. and Gibbs, J. (1981). Brain-gut peptides and the control of food intake. *In* "Neurosecretion and Brain Peptides: Implications for Brain Function and Neurologic Disease" (J. B. Martin and K. Bick, eds), (pp. 389–395). Raven Press, New York.

Smith, G. P., Gibbs, J. and Young, R. C. (1974). Cholecystokinin and intestinal satiety in the rat. *Federation Proc.* **33**, 1146–1149.

Smith, G. P., Jerome, C., Eterno, R. and Cushin, B. (1979). Selective gastric vagotomy decreases the satiety effect of cholecystokinin in rat. *Soc for Neuroscience Abstracts* **5**, 224.

Smith, G. P., Jerome, C., Cushin, B. J., Eterno, R. and Simansky, K. J. (1981). Abdominal vagotomy blocks the satiety effect of cholecystokinin in the rat. *Science* **213**, 1036–1037.

Stricker, E. M. Rowland, N., Saller, C. F. and Friedman, M. I. (1977). Homeostasis during hypoglycemia: central control of adrenal secretion and peripheral control of feeding. *Science* **196**, 79–81.

Stunkard, A. J., Van Itallie, T. B. and Reis, B. B. (1955). The mechanism of satiety: Effect of glucagon on gastric hunger contractions in man. *Proc. Soc. Exp. Biol. Med.* **89**, 258–261.

Thomas, D. W. and Mayer, J. (1968). Meal taking and regulation of food intake by normal and hypothalamic hyperphagic rats. *J. Comp Physiol. Psychol.* **66**. 642–653.

Towbin, E. J. (1955). Thirst and hunger behavior in normal dogs and the effects of vagotomy and sympathectomy. *Am. J. Physiol.* **182**, 337–382.

Vander-Gugten, J., De Kloet, E. R., Versteeg, D. H. G. and Slangen, J. L. (1977). Regional hypothalamic catecholamine metabolism and food intake regulation in the rat. *Brain Res.* **135**, 325–336.

Vanderweele, D. A., Geiselman, P. J. and Novin, D. (1979). Pancreatic glucagon, food deprivation and feeding in intact and vagotomized rabbits. *Physiol. Behav.* **23**, 155–158.

Vanderweele, D. A., Pi-Sunyer, F. X., Novin, D. and Bush, M. J. (1980). Chronic insulin infusion suppresses food ingestion and body weight gain in rats. *Brain Res. Bull.* **5**, Suppl. 4, 7–11.

Walsh, L. L. and Grossman, S. P. (1975). Loss of feeding in response to 2-deoxy-D-glucose but not insulin after zona incerta lesions in the rat. *Physiol. Behav.* **15**, 481–485.

Weiskrantz, L. and Baltzer, V. (1975). Body weight, short-term satiation and the response to reward magnitude shifts. *Quart. J. exptl. Psychol.* **27**, 73–91.

Weiskrantz, L. and Cowey, A. (1963). The aetiology of food reward in monkeys. *Anim. Behav.* **11**, 225–234.

Wiepkema, P. R. (1971). Positive feedbacks at work during feeding. *Behaviour* **39**, 266–273.

Wise, R. A., Spindler, J., de Wit, H. and Gerber, G. J. (1978). Neuroleptic-induced "anhedonia" in rats: pimozide blocks reward quality of food. *Science* **201**, 262–264.

Woods, S. C. and McKay, L. D. (1978). Intraventricular alloxan eliminates feeding elicited by 2-deoxyglucose. *Science* **202**, 1209–1221.

Yamagishi, T. and Debas, H. T. (1978). Cholecystokinin inhibits gastric emptying by acting on both proximal stomach and pylorus. *Am. J. Physiol.* **234**, E375–E378.

Young, R. C., Gibbs, J., Antin, J., Holt, J. and Smith, G. P. (1974). Absence of satiety during sham feeding in the rat. *J. Comp. Physiol. Psychol.* **87**, 795–800.

# 2 □ Neuropharmacology of Feeding

R. Samanin and S. Garattini

## I. INTRODUCTION

There is considerable evidence that most available anorectic drugs depress feeding by changing the activity of central neurons containing putative neurotransmitters such as dopamine, noradrenaline and serotonin. The few drugs found to stimulate appetite might also act by changing the functional activity of these brain substances, although much less is known about this aspect of the problem.

Other brain substances such as gamma-aminobutyric acid (GABA), acetylcholine or enkephalins have been implicated as being important in the regulation of feeding (Kelly *et al.*, 1979; Baile, 1974; Grandison and Guidotti, 1977) but these findings will not be discussed further as there is no evidence currently available on whether such transmitter substances mediate drug-induced changes of feeding behaviour. The catecholamines and serotonin are well represented in the periphery, and some authors suggest peripheral adrenaline and serotonin are involved in anorexia (Russek *et al.*, 1968; Bray and York, 1972). Information on this topic is also limited, and the contribution of these substances to drug effects on feeding is unknown.

In this chapter, the significance of the actions of drugs on brain catecholamines and serotonin will be discussed in relation to their effects on feeding.

## II. THE EFFECT OF DRUGS AFFECTING FEEDING ON CENTRAL DOPAMINE ACTIVITY

### A. Amphetamine

Amphetamine releases dopamine (DA) from nerve endings and inhibits its reuptake into the neurons (Garattini *et al.*, 1978; Garattini and Samanin, 1976). Various studies suggest that these effects mediate the locomotor stimulation and stereotyped movements caused by amphetamine in several animal species. The evidence is derived mainly from the fact that selective destruction of central dopaminergic neurons or treatment with DA antagonists prevents amphetamine-induced motor behaviour (Creese and Iversen, 1973; Fibiger *et al.*, 1973). The overstimulation caused by increased dopaminergic function has made it difficult to assess whether dopamine is involved in amphetamine anorexia as well. The main difficulty resides in the fact that maximal anorexia is usually obtained in animals with doses causing stereotyped movements; such movements themselves can obviously interfere with eating. Furthermore, in keeping with the view that the DA-mediated effects of amphetamine are more closely linked to motor behaviour than to eating, is the observation that DA antagonists completely prevent the effect of amphetamine on motor behaviour, whereas they only partially counteract the depression of feeding (Samanin *et al.*, 1978; Quattrone *et al.*, 1977). This view is supported by the recent finding that it is only the effect of higher doses of amphetamine on feeding which are attenuated by the relatively specific DA receptor blocking drug pimozide; the anorectic effect of lower doses of amphetamine remained unaffected by pimozide (Burridge and Blundell, 1979).

Difficulties in interpreting the changes of dopaminergic activity in relation to feeding behaviour also arise from findings that relatively low doses of apomorphine, a dopamine agonist, either enhance or depress feeding depending on whether the animals are satiated or food-deprived (Eichler and Antelman, 1977). This biphasic action, also observed with amphetamine (Blundell and Latham, 1978), is reminiscent of the inverted U pattern found with the effects of stimulants on various behavioural performances and may well be the consequence of the behavioural arousal and sensory–motor activation caused by an increase in central dopaminergic mechanisms. That changes in central dopamine-dependent sensory–motor mechanisms may lead to dramatic changes in feeding is indicated by recent evidence that the "classical" aphagia induced in rats by lesions of the lateral hypothalamus is in all probability due to a sensory neglect caused by the destruction of dopamine-containing fibres passing through this area (Marshall *et al.*, 1974). The fact that dopamine agonists with less tendency to cause stereotyped movements such as amineptine do not induce anorexia in animals or man also argues against a role of DA in feeding (Samanin *et al.*, 1977a).

A specific involvement of dopamine in feeding regulation has been suggested by Leibowitz who noted depression of feeding on injecting dopamine directly into the perifornical area of the hypothalamus (Leibowitz and Rossakis, 1979). The specificity and physiological significance of this effect, however, are debatable for the following reasons:

(1) Activation of sites sensitive to noradrenaline, adrenaline, serotonin and GABA in this area also depress feeding (Leibowitz and Rossakis, 1978a, 1979; Lehr and Goldman, 1973; Leibowitz, 1978; Kelly *et al.*, 1979).

(2) The effect of dopamine is scarcely altered by pimozide, which is a very potent dopamine receptor blocker (Leibowitz and Rossakis, 1979). It is curious that haloperidol, fluphenazine, chlorpromazine and pimozide prevent the action of dopamine with the same order of potency with which they block the effect of adrenaline (Leibowitz and Rossakis, 1978a, 1979). These data suggest that, as in some peripheral regions, dopamine activates beta adrenergic sites in this hypothalamic area.

(3) The effect on feeding was obtained with a quantity of dopamine (about

10 $\mu$g) well above that contained in the whole brain. Considering that dopamine is poorly represented in the perifornical region (Palkowitz et al., 1974), it is difficult to establish the extent to which this large amount of administered dopamine mimics the effect of endogenously released amine.

(4) The action of dopamine was studied in animals treated with an inhibitor of monoamine oxidase activity (Leibowitz and Rossakis, 1979). The explanation offered for the use of this compound was that in its absence, dopamine is much less effective because it is rapidly metabolized (Leibowitz and Rossakis, 1979). This argument unfortunately does not appear very convincing since membrane uptake is believed to play a major role in terminating the action of amines at postsynaptic receptors (Iversen, 1975) and the rate at which catabolism removes the exogenously administered amine is difficult to estimate. It should instead be considered that monoamine oxidase inhibition could reduce the metabolic degradation of other amines present in this area, thus making it difficult to assess their relative contribution to the final effect.

Although dopamine's role in the physiological regulation of feeding may be questionable, the amine may well be involved in feeding changes observed in certain conditions such as hyperphagia caused by tail-pinch in rats (Antelman and Szechtman, 1975). This form of stress elicits other forms of goal-directed behaviour (Antelman and Caggiula, 1977), in addition to feeding, suggesting that behavioural arousal is the main precipitant of the consumatory response observed in this situation. In view of some behavioural similarities between tail-pinch stress and intracranial stimulation at the lateral hypothalamus, it has been suggested (Valenstein, 1976, 1977) that both conditions give rise to a form of "neurotic" behaviour rather than one motivated by nutritional needs or other biological deficits. It is of interest that the behavioural responses in both conditions are blocked by central dopamine antagonists (Antelman and Caggiula, 1977; Phillips and Nikaido, 1975).

In discussing the role of dopamine in the action of amphetamine, it should be mentioned that dopamine has been implicated in central motivational and/or reinforcement processes as well as in the reinforcing properties shown by amphetamine in various species (Fibiger and Phillips, 1979). That these effects are separate from those on motor behaviour is indicated by the fact that pimozide attenuates lever-pressing and running for food reward in hungry rats at doses which do not cause incapacitating sedation or motor effects (Wise et al., 1978). The increased rate of responding for intravenous amphetamine in rats after pimozide injection has also been interpreted as a consequence of reduced reinforcing properties of amphetamine after dopamine receptor blockade (Yokel and Wise, 1976). It is therefore possible that changes of dopaminergic activity modify feeding by changing the reward quality of food and/or how often eating takes place. This could help explain the increase in feeding observed with long-term neuroleptic treatment which raises the number and sensitivity of central dopamine receptors (Burt et al., 1977).

In conclusion, moderate activation of dopaminergic function induced by low doses of amphetamine results in increased locomotor activity and enhances many behavioural performances in various species. The reinforcing properties of amphetamine appear to depend on brain dopamine as well. Dopamine is involved in the euphoric effects and addictive properties of amphetamine in humans since dopamine receptor blockers markedly reduce them (Gunne, 1977). Amphetamine-induced anorexia in humans, however, is not affected by pimozide (Silverstone, 1978). The stereotyped movements and excitation syndrome found after high doses of amphetamine also appear to depend on dopaminergic mechanisms in the brain. Although a physiological role of dopamine in the regulation of feeding is not clearly established, changes in dopamine function can alter feeding behaviour by modifying the reinforcing and motivational qualities of food. The changes in feeding occurring during long-term treatment with neuroleptics (Robinson et al., 1975a, b) may partially be explained on this basis. It is of interest that this type of hyperphagia is resistant to amphetamine treatment but is reduced by fenfluramine (Jensen and Kirk, 1972) a drug believed to depress feeding by increasing serotonin function (Garattini et al., 1979). Fenfluramine has been shown recently to block the stimulatory effects of amphetamine probably by indirectly inhibiting dopamine-containing neurons in the brain (Bendotti et al., 1980).

It has been suggested (Antelman and Caggiula, 1977) that, like tail-pinch feeding in rats, stress-induced eating in humans such as "reactive obesity" and "night eating syndrome" described respectively by Bruch (1957, 1973) and Stunkard (1955) involves increased dopaminergic function. An elevated dopaminergic tone might also contribute to the increased sensitivity of obese patients to environmental, food-related cues, described by Schachter (1968). Although only speculative, these suggestions imply that drugs activating central serotonin transmission might be the drugs of choice in these conditions.

## B. Mazindol and Diethylpropion

These drugs, like amphetamine, cause central stimulation (Garattini et al., 1978; Garattini and Samanin, 1976). This effect depends on central dopaminergic mechanisms since it is blocked by treatment with dopamine receptor blockers (Carruba et al., 1978; Offermeier and du Preez, 1978; Borsini et al., 1979; Garattini and Samanin, 1976). The effects of mazindol and diethylpropion on motor behaviour are blocked by drugs interfering with the synthesis and storage of brain dopamine (Carruba et al., 1978; Offermeier and du Preez, 1978) indicating that presynaptic dopamine mechanisms are mainly affected. This has been confirmed by biochemical studies (Garattini et al., 1978; Carruba et al., 1978; Offermeier and du Preez, 1978). Regarding the effects on food intake, the effect of mazindol, but not that of diethylpropion, is partially prevented by procedures which reduce central dopaminergic activity (Borsini et al., 1979; Samanin et al., 1977b). Mazindol, however, is more potent than diethylpropion on dopaminergic mechanisms and motor behaviour (Garattini et al., 1978). Thus, as in the case of amphetamine, excessive motor stimulation may partially be responsible for the blockade of feeding caused by this compound in rats.

In this respect, although mazindol has a chemical structure different from that of phenylethylamine, it is very similar to amphetamine, whereas diethylpropion, a phenylethylamine, appears to be quantitatively and qualitatively different. This may explain the less addictive properties of diethylpropion in man (Hoekenga *et al.*, 1978).

## C. Fenfluramine

This drug affects dopamine mechanisms in the brain quite differently from the drugs discussed above (Garattini *et al.*, 1974, 1975a, b). At doses higher than those causing reduction of food intake, fenfluramine increases the metabolism of brain dopamine (Garattini *et al.*, 1974, 1975b). However, it does not cause motor stimulation or stereotyped movements and can even reduce the stimulatory effects of amphetamine (Garattini *et al.*, 1975a; Bendotti *et al.*, 1980).

Since the effect of fenfluramine on dopamine metabolism is prevented by direct dopamine agonists such as apomorphine and piribedil, it was suggested that fenfluramine acts on brain dopamine through a mechanism similar to that of neuroleptics (Jori *et al.*, 1974). These drugs are purported to increase striatal dopamine metabolism through a feedback mechanism following receptor blockade (Da Prada and Pletscher, 1966). Further studies, however, have shown that fenfluramine, unlike neuroleptics, does not displace dopamine binding at brain membranes (Burt *et al.*, 1976) indicating that mechanisms other than postsynaptic dopamine receptor blockade may be responsible for the changes of dopamine metabolism. It has been recently suggested that the effect of the *d*-isomer of fenfluramine on striatal dopamine metabolism is mediated by its ability to activate serotoninergic function in the brain since the effect is blocked by drugs which prevent fenfluramine's action on brain serotonin (Crunelli *et al.*, 1980). This, however, does not apply to the *l*-isomer whose effects on dopamine metabolism are not affected by drugs acting on serotonin (Crunelli *et al.*, 1980).

Unlike the *d*-isomer, *l*-fenfluramine may act by changing the intraneuronal disposition of dopamine (Bendotti *et al.*, 1980). Considering that *in vivo d*- and *l*-fenfluramine form their respective de-ethylated metabolites which also have different effects on central serotonin and dopamine (Garattini *et al.*, 1979), the exact mechanism by which fenfluramine interacts with the dopaminergic system is difficult to define. Reduced dopaminergic function rather than activation of the dopaminergic mechanism appears however to be the overall effect of fenfluramine. The limited tendency among patients to abuse fenfluramine (Estrada, 1979; Gotestam, 1979) may partially depend on the drug's inability to cause central dopaminergic activation.

## III. THE EFFECT OF DRUGS AFFECTING FEEDING ON CENTRAL NORADRENALINE ACTIVITY

### A. Amphetamine

Amphetamine releases noradrenaline from presynaptic nerve terminals and inhibits its reuptake into the neuron (Garattini *et al.*, 1978; Garattini and

Samanin, 1976). It also increases the turnover of brain noradrenaline and the level of its O-methylmetabolite (Garattini and Samanin, 1976) thus increasing noradrenaline availability at post-synaptic receptors. When given systemically, amphetamine causes anorexia as its main effect (Garattini and Samanin, 1976), but it can also stimulate feeding when administered at very low doses (Dobrzanski and Doggett, 1976). There is evidence that both of these effects depend on its action on brain noradrenaline, although the type and distribution of the adrenergic sites mediating these effects can be different. Increased feeding has been noted on injecting amphetamine in the medial part of the hypothalamus, particularly the paraventricular nucleus, and this effect is inhibited by alpha-adrenergic blockers (Leibowitz, 1976). The same effect is seen on injecting noradrenaline in this area. Since feeding can be elicited by applying noradrenaline in other brain areas (Lytle, 1977) and noradrenaline released by amphetamine is a widespread phenomenon in the central nervous system, other brain areas may also be involved in amphetamine-induced feeding.

At low doses, amphetamine increases spontaneous locomotor activity and many behavioural performances, and these effects appear to be partially mediated by its effect on noradrenaline (Maj et al., 1972; Schoot, van der et al., 1962). It has been suggested (Fibiger and Phillips, 1979) that by releasing catecholamines in the brain, amphetamine at low doses raises the general level of arousal and/or motivation and consequently the probability of specific behavioural patterns occurring. This would be more in line with the fact that low doses of amphetamine enhance many behavioural outputs, including feeding.

As stated above, depression of feeding is commonly observed after moderate doses of amphetamine (about 1–2 mg/kg in rats). It has been suggested that amphetamine depresses feeding by activating beta-adrenergic and dopaminergic sites in the perifornical area of the hypothalamus (Leibowitz and Rossakis, 1978b) because the reduction of food intake caused by local application of amphetamine in this area is prevented by dopamine and beta-adrenergic blockers (Leibowitz and Rossakis, 1978b). As in the case of dopamine, amphetamine effects were obtained by injecting 50–100 nmol of the drug, much more than that found in the whole brain after systemic injection of a dose causing maximal anorexia (Jori et al., 1978; Garattini et al., 1975c) thus casting doubt on the significance of these findings in interpreting the action of systemically administered amphetamine.

That central noradrenergic neurons are involved in the anorectic activity of amphetamine is suggested by the fact that selective lesions of noradrenergic fibres passing through the so-called ventral noradrenergic bundle (VNB) completely prevent amphetamine affecting food intake (Ahlskog, 1974; Borsini et al., 1979; Samanin et al., 1977b). Of interest is the fact that this lesion does not prevent the drug acting on motor behaviour (Quattrone et al., 1977) arguing in favour of a specific role of this system in amphetamine anorexia. These findings disprove the assumption that amphetamine anorexia is closely associated with its stimulatory effects. The importance of the ventral noradrenergic bundle for the regulation of feeding is clearly shown by the hyperphagia and obesity that develop after lesions in this area (Ahlskog, 1974).

It has been suggested that destruction of noradrenergic terminals of this system significantly contribute to the hyperphagia and obesity observed after lesions made in the medial hypothalamus, although various differences between the two differently induced forms of hyperphagia have been noted. This however does not disprove a contribution of the VNB to hyperphagia caused by hypothalamic lesions since such lesions are likely to cause destruction of other neuronal elements which can qualitatively and quantitatively change the effect of VNB nerve terminal degeneration (Marshall, 1976). Some authors (Cox and Maickel, 1975) doubt that amphetamine anorexia is mediated by central noradrenergic mechanisms since treatment with alpha-methyl-paratyrosine (alpha MpT), a blocker of catecholamine synthesis, completely prevents the stimulatory action with little effect on the reduction of food intake. In addition, dopamine beta hydroxylase inhibitors, which selectively block noradrenaline synthesis, hardly affect amphetamine anorexia (Franklin and Herberg, 1977), thus also apparently confuting noradrenaline involvement.

It should, however, be considered that, while the amphetamine-induced release of dopamine closely depends on synthesis of the amine (Van Rossum et al., 1962), the mechanism of noradrenaline release appears to involve removal of the amine from a larger pool less dependent on amine synthesis (Engberg and Svensson, 1979). This difference is illustrated by the fact that reserpine, which preferentially affects catecholamine storage, significantly counteracts the anorectic activity but not the stimulatory effects of amphetamine (Schmitt, 1973; Neill and Grossman, 1971). Furthermore, in keeping with this hypothesis, amphetamine at relatively high doses causes marked depletion of brain noradrenaline with little effect on dopamine (Garattini et al., 1975a). Thus, the data with alpha MpT and dopamine beta-hydroxylase inhibitors do not disprove that noradrenaline mediates the effect of amphetamine on food intake.

It has been found that adrenaline-containing fibres run with noradrenergic fibres in the VNB (Hokfelt et al., 1974) and adrenaline depresses feeding when injected in the perifornical area (Antelman and Szechtman, 1975). Since most procedures and drugs used to affect noradrenergic mechanisms also act on brain adrenaline, the relative roles of these brain amines in amphetamine anorexia are difficult to disentangle.

Hyperphagia has been described in monkeys after lesions of the locus coeruleus, an area rich in noradrenergic neurons (Redmond et al., 1977). Although no direct evidence was offered that this hyperphagia was due to selective degeneration of noradrenergic neurons, it was suggested that these neurons might constitute a central adrenergic satiety mechanism (Redmond et al., 1977). However, the locus coeruleus is not involved in the depression of food intake caused by amphetamine in rats (Quattrone et al., 1977). In view of the fact that it is involved in the mechanism of arousal and wakefulness (Jouvet, 1974; Fuxe et al., 1974) and that noradrenergic neurons arising in this area facilitate dopaminergic function in the brain (Pycock *et al.*, 1975; Anden and Grabowska, 1976), it is more likely that part of the stimulatory effects of amphetamine depend on its ability to release noradrenaline from terminals of neurons originating in this brain area.

In conclusion, the bulk of data suggests that amphetamine causes anorexia by releasing noradrenaline (and/or adrenaline) from fibres in the so-called ventral noradrenergic bundle whose cells of origins are in the medulla oblongata and which innervates various forebrain areas, including the hypothalamus. Whether the postsynaptic sites involve beta-adrenergic receptors (as suggested by studies using intracerebral injections) is difficult to establish since systemic administration of beta-adrenergic blockers do not normally counteract amphetamine anorexia (Garattini and Samanin, 1976).

Other noradrenergic neurons, together with dopaminergic neurons, may be involved in some aspects of behavioural activation, including feeding, elicited by very low doses of amphetamine.

## B. Other Drugs

Mazindol and diethylpropion activate central noradrenergic mechanisms (Garattini and Samanin, 1976; Carruba *et al.*, 1978; Offermeier and du Preez, 1978). Although some authors have favoured an involvement of brain dopamine in the anorectic activity of mazindol (Carruba *et al.*, 1978), the effects on noradrenaline appear to be necessary for mazindol and diethylpropion to depress food intake as shown by the fact that lesions of the VNB completely prevent the anorectic activity of these drugs (Borsini *et al.*, 1979; Samanin *et al.*, 1977b).

Fenfluramine increases the release of noradrenaline and its metabolism in the brain (Calderini *et al.*, 1975) with a mechanism different from that of amphetamine. Fenfluramine releases noradrenaline mainly at the intraneuronal level with most amine catabolized by monoamine oxidases before leaving the nerve terminals (Ziance and Rutledge, 1972), while amphetamine releases it directly in the extraneuronal space (Garattini and Samanin, 1976). It cannot be excluded however that fenfluramine to some extent activates adrenergic mechanisms in intact animals, since marked sympathetic effects have been described after its administration (Lake *et al.*, 1979).

## IV. THE EFFECT OF DRUGS AFFECTING FEEDING ON CENTRAL SEROTONIN ACTIVITY

## A. Fenfluramine

There is considerable evidence that serotonin plays an important role in the reduction of food intake induced by fenfluramine. Fenfluramine releases serotonin from nerve endings and inhibits its reuptake into the neuron (Garattini and Samanin, 1976; Garattini *et al.*, 1975b). The mechanism by which it releases 5HT may differ according to whether the parent drug or its main metabolite, norfenfluramine, is given. Reserpine pretreatment prevents the effect of d-fenfluramine (dF) on 5HT release but potentiates the effect of d-norfenfluramine (dNF) (Mennini et al., 1981) suggesting that these compounds normally release 5HT from two different pools. The effects of l-fenfluramine and l-norfenfluramine are less altered by reserpine treatment (Mennini et al., 1981). Since both isomers and their metabolites are involved when the racemic form of fenfluramine is administered (Garattini et al., 1979), their differential effects on serotonin release must be taken into account when interpreting the functional effects observed with fenfluramine.

The following findings suggest that serotonin is involved in the anorectic activity of fenfluramine:

(1) Destruction of 5HT neurons prevents fenfluramine anorexia (Samanin et al., 1972; Clineschmidt et al., 1974).

(2) Fenfluramine anorexia is counteracted by treatment with 5HT antagonists (Garattini and Samanin, 1976).

(3) Inhibitors of 5HT uptake mechanism which prevent the effect of fenfluramine on brain serotonin, significantly reduce its effect on food intake (Garattini and Samanin, 1976; Garattini et al., 1975a; Garattini et al., 1974; Garattini et al., 1975b).

Although some authors have found a reduction of fenfluramine anorexia in animals injected intracerebrally with 5, 6 dihydroxytryptamine (Clineschmidt et al., 1974) which is neurotoxic for central 5HT neurons (Nobin and Bjorklund, 1978), other authors using 5, 7 dihydroxytryptamine (57HT), which also causes depletion of brain 5HT (Nobin and Bjorklund, 1978) have found no effect or even a potentiation of fenfluramine's effect on food intake (Hoebel et al., 1978). These latter authors suggest that fenfluramine acts at postsynaptic 5HT receptors or through mechanisms other than 5HT. The first hypothesis is not likely since fenfluramine is a very poor displacer of $^3$H5HT binding at brain membranes (Garattini et al., 1979). In view of the ample evidence of 5HT's involvement in fenfluramine anorexia, a possible explanation of 57HT's failure to affect fenfluramine anorexia in rats is its relative ineffectiveness in causing 5HT depletion in certain brain areas (Nobin and Bjorklund, 1978). The integrity of an area close to the pons-mesencephalon raphe nuclei has been shown to be crucial for the anorectic activity of fenfluramine in rats (Samanin et al., 1972) and the brainstem is particularly resistant to the action of 57HT on serotonin (Nobin and Bjorklund, 1978).

Another serotonin-dependent effect of fenfluramine is its ability to reduce food intake by sparing protein consumption (Wurtman and Wurtman, 1977), as shown by the fact that drugs enhancing 5HT-transmission reduce carbohydrate consumption (Wurtman and Wurtman, 1979) while depletion of brain 5HT selectively reduces protein intake in rats (Ashley et al., 1979). Amphetamine, on the other hand, reduces protein and caloric intake proportionally (Wurtman and Wurtman, 1977). Another interesting difference between these drugs is that fenfluramine blocks hyperphagia induced in rats by tail pinch, whereas amphetamine has no such effect (Antelman et al., 1979).

This effect of fenfluramine appears to be mediated by its action on 5HT since it is also observed with direct 5HT agonists (Antelman *et al.*, 1979). These findings are of interest in view of the suggested similarities between hyperphagia induced by tail pinch stress in rats and some forms of excessive eating in humans (Antelman *et al.*, 1979).

On the basis of some differences noted between fenfluramine and amphetamine in changing particular aspects of feeding such as onset of feeding, meal size, rate of eating, etc., it has been suggested (Blundell *et al.*, 1976) that fenfluramine is primarily involved in satiety mechanisms, while amphetamine acts mainly by reducing hunger. No convincing evidence has been provided however in support of this hypothesis and some of the different effects of the two drugs may well be explained by their different kinetics and/or general effects on behaviour (sedation *vs* stimulation). At this stage of knowledge, it is much safer merely to say that fenfluramine depresses feeding by a mechanism which is different in many respects from that of amphetamine. That brain serotonin normally inhibits feeding is shown by the increase in feeding which results from the intracerebral injection of 5HT depletors such as parachlorophenylalanine, PCPA or 57HT, or systemic injection of 5HT antagonists (Breisch *et al.*, 1976; Saller and Stricker, 1976; Blundell, 1977). However, as in the case of catecholamines, serotonin may affect many central functions, as shown by the many types of behaviour affected by changes in serotonin transmission. Therefore, it has still to be determined whether the increase of feeding obtained by reducing serotonin transmission in the whole brain is due to a general disinhibitory effect on behaviour or specifically involves mechanisms regulating satiety and hunger. Depression of feeding has been seen when serotonin is applied directly in the hypothalamus (Leibowitz and Rossakis, 1979) but the reservations expressed about this approach when discussing the effect of drugs on catecholamine pathways apply equally to serotonin pathways. Obviously, further studies are needed to clarify the exact mechanism by which changes in serotonin actively affect feeding.

## B. Piperazine Derivatives

In agreement with the hypothesis that increased central serotonin transmission causes anorexia, recent findings show that quipazine, a central serotonin agonist (Samanin *et al.*, 1980) markedly depresses food intake in rats, and metergoline, a serotonin antagonist, completely prevents this effect (Samanin *et al.*, 1977c). Part of quipazine's effect on feeding may derive from its ability to release serotonin from nerve terminals since lesions of central serotoninergic neurons partially prevent its reducing food intake (Samanin *et al.*, 1978). Drugs interfering with catecholamines do not modify quipazine's effect (Samanin *et al.*, 1978). More recently, metachlorophenylpiperazine (mCPP), a potent central 5HT agonist, was also shown to reduce food intake by acting on brain serotonin (Samanin *et al.*, 1979). Since its effect was not modified by destruction of central serotonin-containing neurons, but was prevented by 5HT antagonists, mCPP's ability to mimic serotonin at postsynaptic receptors is considered of major importance for its anorectic activity (Samanin *et al.*, 1979).

Another piperazine derivative has been recently shown to depress feeding in rats and cats (Clineschmidt *et al.*, 1977). Since this drug shows no affinity for serotonin binding sites *in vitro* (Fuller *et al.*, 1978) it may depress feeding by a presynaptic mechanism. Recent studies on the mechanism by which feeding is depressed by drugs acting on serotonin show that increased serotonin release and/or direct stimulation of postsynaptic receptors are more important in mediating drug-induced anorexia than other mechanisms such as uptake inhibition (Samanin *et al.*, 1980).

Although serotonin's exact role in the regulation of feeding is not known, it can be concluded that drugs enhancing central serotonin transmission reduce food intake without causing gross behavioural changes. Increased feeding has also been observed in conditions in which serotonin function was assumed to be reduced (Blundell, 1977), although the relative specificity and effectiveness of blocking central serotonin receptors with available drugs make the relation between reduction of serotonin function and increase of feeding less certain. The development of more selective, centrally effective serotonin antagonists may help considerably in assessing its role in regulating feeding and to what extent blocking its function may stimulate appetite.

## C. Other Drugs

At high doses, amphetamine can increase the synthesis of brain serotonin (Reid, 1970), but it is not clear whether this effect is a primary one or is secondary to other actions in the central nervous system. Mazindol is a potent inhibitor of serotonin uptake (Garattini *et al.*, 1978; Garattini and Samanin, 1976) while diethylpropion has little effect on serotonin mechanisms in the brain (Garattini *et al.*, 1978). The effects of amphetamine and mazindol on brain serotonin do not significantly contribute to their anorectic activity since neither destruction of central serotonin-containing neurons nor treatment with serotonin antagonists prevents their action on food intake (Garattini and Samanin, 1976).

## V. CONCLUDING REMARKS

On examining the effects of drugs known to suppress feeding in laboratory animals and man, the following conclusions can be drawn:

(A) The anorectic activity of amphetamine, mazindol and diethylpropion depends mainly, if not exclusively, on their ability to release noradrenaline (and/or adrenaline) from central neurons associated with the so-called ventral noradrenergic bundle. This system appears to be specifically involved in feeding suppression since the stimulatory effects of these compounds are not prevented by destruction of this area. Some aspects of amphetamine's stimu-

latory action may involve noradrenergic neurons other than those in the VNB.
(B) Brain dopamine is mainly involved in the behavioural stimulation caused
by amphetamine, mazindol and, to a lesser degree, diethylpropion. In spite of
various suggestions of dopamine involvement in feeding, its role in drug-
induced anorexia is doubtful.
(C) Drugs such as fenfluramine and some piperazine derivatives depress
feeding by releasing serotonin from central neurons and/or mimicking its
action on postsynaptic receptors. These drugs have little effect on catecholamines or act upon them differently from amphetamine. The lack of central
stimulatory effects may be due to their inability to activate catecholaminergic
mechanisms in the brain.

# REFERENCES

Ahlskog, J. E. (1974). Food intake and amphetamine anorexia after selective forebrain
    norepinephrine loss. *Brain Res.* **82**, 211–240.
Andén, N. E. and Grabowska, M. (1976). Pharmacological evidence for a stimulation of
    dopamine neurons by noradrenaline neurons in the brain. *Eur. J. Pharmac.* **39**,
    275–282.
Antelman, S. M. and Caggiula, A. R. (1977). Tails of stress-related behavior: A
    neuropharmacological analysis. *In* "Animal Models in Psychiatry and Neurology" (I.
    Hanin and E. Usdin, eds), pp. 227–245. Pergamon Press, Oxford.
Antelman, S. M., Caggiula, A. R., Eichler, A. J. and Lucik, R. R. (1979). The
    importance of stress in assessing the effects of anorectic drugs. *Curr. Med. Res.
    Opinion* **6**, suppl. 1, 73–82.
Antelman, S. M. and Szechtman, H. (1975). Tail-pinch induces eating in sated rats
    which appears to depend on nigrostriatal dopamine. *Science* **189**, 731–733.
Ashley, D. V. M., Coscina, D. V. and Anderson, G. H. (1979). Selective decrease in
    protein intake following brain serotonin depletion. *Life Sci.* **24**, 973–984.
Baile, C. A. (1974). Putative neurotransmitters in the hypothalamus and feeding. *Fed.
    Proc.* **33**, 1166–1175.
Bendotti, C., Borsini, F., Zanini, M. G., Samanin, R. and Garattini, S. (1980). Effect of
    fenfluramine and norfenfluramine stereoisomers on stimulant effects of d-ampheta-
    mine and apomorphine in the rat. *Pharmac. Res. Commun.* **12**, 567–574.
Blundell, J. E. (1977). Is there a role for serotonin (5-hydroxy-tryptamine) in feeding?
    *Int. J. Obesity* **1**, 15–42.
Blundell, J. E. and Latham, C. J. (1978). Pharmacological manipulation of feeding
    behavior: Possible influences of serotonin and dopamine on food intake. *In* "Central
    Mechanisms of Anorectic Drugs, (S. Garattini and R. Samanin, eds)" pp. 83–109.
    Raven Press, New York.
Blundell, J. E., Latham, C. J. and Leshem, M. B. (1976). Differences between the
    anorexic actions of amphetamine and fenfluramine: Possible effects on hunger and
    satiety. *J. Pharm. Pharmac.* **28**, 471–477.
Borsini, F., Bendotti, C., Carli, M., Poggesi, E. and Samanin, R. (1979). The roles of
    brain noradrenaline and dopamine in the anorectic activity of diethylpropion in rats.
    A comparison with d-amphetamine. *Res. Commun. Chem. Pathol. Pharmac.* **26**,
    3–11.
Bray, G. A. and York, D. A. (1972). Studies on food intake of genetically obese rats.

*Amer. J. Physiol.* **223**, 176–179.

Breisch, S. T., Zemlan, F. P. and Hoebel, B. G. (1976). Hyperphagia and obesity following serotonin depletion by intraventricular p-chlorophenylalanine. *Science* **192**, 382–385.

Bruch, H. (1957). "The Importance of Overweight". Norton, New York.

Bruch, H. (1973). "Eating Disorders". Basic Books, New York.

Burridge, S. B. and Blundell, J. E. (1979). Amphetamine anorexia: antagonism by typical but not atypical neuroleptics. *Neuropharmacology* **18**, 453–457.

Burt, D. R., Creese, I. and Snyder, S. H. (1976). Properties of [³H]-haloperidol and [³H] dopamine binding associated with dopamine receptors in calf brain membranes. *Molec. Pharmac.* **12**, 800–812.

Burt, D. R., Creese, I. and Snyder, S. H. (1977). Antischizophrenic drugs: Chronic treatment elevates dopamine receptor binding in brain. *Science* **196**, 326–328.

Calderini, G., Morselli, P. L. and Garattini, S. (1975). Effect of amphetamine and fenfluramine on brain noradrenaline and Mopeg SO . *Eur. J. Pharmac.* **34**, 345–350.

Carruba, M. O., Zambotti, F., Vicentini, L., Picotti, G. B. and Mantegazza, P. (1978). Pharmacology and biochemical profile of a new anorectic drug: Mazindol. *In* "Central Mechanisms of Anorectic Drugs" (S. Garattini and R. Samanin, eds), pp. 145–164. Raven Press, New York.

Clineschmidt, B. V., Hanson, H. M., Pflueger, A. B. and McGuffin, J. C. (1977). Anorexigenic and ancillary actions of MK-212 (6-chloro-2-[1-piperazinyl]-pyrazine; CPP). *Psychopharmacology* **55**, 27–33.

Clineschmidt, B. V., McGuffin, J. C. and Werner, A. B. (1974). Role of monoamines in the anorexigenic actions of fenfluramine, amphetamine and p-chloromethamphetamine. *Eur. J. Pharmac.* **27**, 313–323.

26.

Cox, R. H. Jr and Maickel, R. P. (1975). Differential effects of αMT on anorectic and stimulatory action of amphetamines. *Res. Commun. Chem. Pathol. Pharmac.* **12**, 621–626.

Creese, I. and Iversen, S. D. (1973). Blockage of amphetamine induced motor stimulation and stereotypy in the adult rat following neonatal treatment with 6-hydroxy-dopamine. *Brain. Res.* **55**, 369–382.

Crunelli, V., Bernasconi, S. and Samanin, R. (1980). Effects of d- and l-fenfluramine on striatal homovanillic acid concentrations in rats after pharmacological manipulation of brain serotonin. *Pharmac. Res. Commun.* **12**, 215–223.

Da Prada, M. and Pletscher, A. (1966). Acceleration of the cerebral dopamine turnover by chlorpromazine. *Experientia* **22**, 465–466.

Dobrzanski, S. and Doggett, N. S. (1976). The effects of (+)-amphetamine and fenfluramine on feeding in starved and satiated mice. *Psychopharmacology* **48**, 283–286.

Eichler, A. J. and Antelman, S. M. (1977). Apomorphine: Feeding or anorexia depending on internal state. *Commun. Psychopharmac.* **1**, 533–540.

Engberg, G. and Svensson, T. H. (1979). Amphetamine-induced inhibition of central noradrenergic neurons: A pharmacological analysis. *Life Sci.* **24**, 2245–2254.

Estrada, U. (1979). Addiction liability of fenfluramine. *Curr. Med. Res. Opinion* **6**, suppl. 1, 118–124.

Fibiger, H. C., Fibiger, H. P. and Zis, A. P. (1973). Attenuation of amphetamine-induced motor stimulation and stereotypy by 6-hydroxy-dopamine in the rat. *Brit. J. Pharmac.* **47**, 683–692.

Fibiger, H. C. and Phillips, A. G. (1979). Dopamine and the neural mechanisms of reinforcement. In "The Neurobiology of Dopamine" (A. S. Horn, J. Korf and B. H. C. Westerink, eds), pp. 597–615. Academic Press, London and New York.

Franklin, K. B. J. and Herberg, L. J. (1977). Amphetamine induces anorexia even after inhibition of noradrenaline synthesis. *Neuropharmacology* **16**, 45–46.

Fuller, R. W., Snoddy, H. D., Mason, N. R. and Molloy, B. B. (1978). Effect of 1-(m-trifluoromethylphenyl)-piperazine on $^3$H-serotonin binding to membranes from rat brain *in vitro* and on serotonin turnover in rat brain *in vivo*. *Eur. J. Pharmac.* **52**, 11–16.

Fuxe, K., Lidbrink, P., Hökfelt, T., Bolme, P. and Goldstein, M. (1974). Effects of piperoxane on sleep and waking in the rat. Evidence for increased waking by blocking inhibitory adrenaline receptors on the locus coeruleus. *Acta Physiol. Scand.* **91**, 566–567.

Garattini, S., Bizzi, A., de Gaetano, G., Jori, A. and Samanin, R. (1975a). Recent advances in the pharmacology of anorectic agents. *In* "Recent Advances in Obesity Research, I" (A. Howard, ed.), pp. 354–367. Newman Publ., London.

Garattini, S., Bonaccorsi, A., Jori, A. and Samanin, R. (1974). Appetite suppressant drugs: past, present and future. *In* "Obesity: Causes, Consequences and Treatment" (L. Lasagna, ed.), pp. 70–80. Medcom Press, New York.

Garattini, S., Borroni, E., Mennini, T. and Samanin, R. (1978). Differences and similarities between anorectic agents. *In* "Central Mechanisms of Anorectic Drugs" (S. Garattini and R. Samanin, eds), pp. 127–143. Raven Press, New York.

Garattini, S., Buczko, W., Jori, A. and Samanin, R. (1975b). On the mechanism of action of fenfluramine. *Postgrad. Med. J.* **51**, suppl. 1, 27–35.

Garattini, S., Caccia, S., Mennini, T., Samanin, R., Consolo, S. and Ladinsky, H. (1979). Notes on the biochemical pharmacology of the anorectic drug fenfluramine. *Curr. Med. Res. Opinion* **6**, suppl. 1, 15–27.

Garattini, S., Jori, A., Manara, L. and Samanin, R. (1975c). 6-Hydroxydopamine, a tool to study distribution of drugs in the catecholaminergic system. *In* "Chemical Tools in Catecholamine Research" Vol. 1. (G. Jonsson, T. Malmfors and Ch. Sachs, eds), pp. 303–309. North Holland, Amsterdam.

Garattini, S. and Samanin, R. (1976). Anorectic drugs and brain neurotransmitters. *In* "Appetite and Food Intake" Dahlem Konferenzen, (T. Silverstone, ed.), pp. 83–108.

Götestam, K. G. (1979). Investigations of abuse potential of anorectic drugs. *Curr. Med. Res. Opinion* **6**, suppl. 1, 125–134.

Grandison, L. and Guidotti, A. (1977). Stimulation of food intake by muscimol and beta endorphin. *Neuropharmacology* **16**, 533–536.

Gunne, L.-M. (1977). Effects of amphetamine in humans. *In* "Handbook of Experimental Pharmacology" Vol. 45 "Drug Addiction II" (W. R. Martin, ed), pp. 247–275. Springer Verlag, Berlin.

Hoebel, B. G., Zemlan, F. P., Trulson, M. E., MacKenzie, R. G., DuCret, R. P. and Norelli, C. (1978). Differential effects of p-chlorophenylalanine and 5,7-dihydroxy-tryptamine on feeding in rats. *Ann. N.Y. Acad. Sci.* **305**, 590–594.

Hoekenga, M. T., Dillon, R. H. and Leyland, H. M. (1978). A comprehensive review of diethylpropion hydrochloride. *In* "Central Mechanisms of Anorectic Drugs" (S. Garattini and R. Samanin, eds), pp. 391–404. Raven Press, New York.

Hökfelt, T., Fuxe, K., Goldstein, M. and Johansson, O. (1974). Immunohistochemical evidence for the existence of adrenaline neurons in the rat brain. *Brain Res.* **66**, 235–251.

Iversen, L. L. (1975). Uptake processes for biogenic amines. *In* "Handbook of Psychopharmacology" Vol. 3 (L. L. Iversen, S. D. Iversen and S. H. Snyder, eds), pp. 381–442, Plenum Press, New York.

Jensen, P. S. and Kirk, L. (1972). Presented at the "Annual Meeting of the Scandinavian Society of Psychopharmacology" Copenhagen.

Jori, A., Caccia, S. and De Ponte, P. (1978). Differences in the availability of d- and l-enantiomers after administration of racemic amphetamine to rats. *Xenobiotica* **8**, 589–595.

Jori, A., Cecchetti, G., Ghezzi, D. and Samanin, R. (1974). Biochemical and behavioral antagonism between fenfluramine and apomorphine in rats. *Eur. J. Pharmac.* **26**, 179–183.

Jouvet, M. (1974). Monoaminergic regulation of the sleep-walking cycle in the cat. *In* "The Neurosciences: Third Study Program" (F. O. Schmitt and F. G. Worden, eds), pp. 499–508. M.I.T. Press, Cambridge.

Kelly, J., Rothstein, J. and Grossman, S. P. (1979). GABA and hypothalamic-feeding systems. *Physiol. Behav.* **23**, 1123–1134.

Lake, C. R., Coleman, M. D., Ziegler, M. G. and Murphy, D. C. (1979). Fenfluramine and its effects on the sympathetic nervous system in man. *Curr. Med. Res. Opinion* **6**, suppl. 1, 63–72.

Lehr, D. and Goldman, W. (1973). Continued pharmacologic analysis of consummatory behavior in the albino rat. *Eur. J. Pharmac.* **23**, 197–210.

Leibowitz, S. F. (1976). Brain catecholaminergic mechanisms for control of hunger. *In* "Hunger: Basic Mechanisms and Clinical Implications" (D. Novin, W. Wyrwicka and G. Bray, eds), pp. 1–18. Raven Press, New York.

Leibowitz, S. F. (1978). Identification of catecholamine receptor mechanisms in the perifornical lateral hypothalamus and their role in mediating amphetamine and L-Dopa anorexia. *In* "Central Mechanisms of Anorectic Drugs" (S. Garattini and R. Samanin, eds), pp. 39–82. Raven Press, New York.

Leibowitz, S. F. and Rossakis, C. (1978a). Pharmacological characterization of perifornical hypothalamic $\beta$-adrenergic receptors mediating feeding inhibition in the rat. *Neuropharmacology* **17**, 691–702.

Leibowitz, S. F. and Rossakis, C. (1978b). Analysis of feeding suppression produced by perifornical hypothalamic injection of catecholamines, amphetamines and mazindol. *Eur. J. Pharmac.* **53**, 69–81.

Leibowitz, S. F. and Rossakis, C. (1979). Pharmacological characterization of perifornical hypothalamic dopamine, receptors mediating feeding inhibition in the rat. *Brain Res.* **172**, 115–130.

Lytle, L. D. (1977). Control of eating behavior. *In* "Nutrition and the Brain" Vol. 2 (R. J. Wurtman and J. J. Wurtman, eds), pp. 1–145. Raven Press, New York.

Maj, J., Sowinska, H., Kapturkiewicz, Z. and Sarnek, J. (1972). The effect of L-dopa and (+)-amphetamine on the locomotor activity after pimozide and phenoxybenzamine. *J. Pharm. Pharmac.* **24**, 412–413.

Marshall, J. F. (1976). Neurochemistry of central monoamine systems as related to food intake. *In* "Appetite and Food Intake", Dahlem Konferenzen, (T. Silverstone, ed.), pp. 43–63.

Marshall, J. F., Richardson, J. S. and Teitelbaum, P. (1974). Nigrostriatal bundle damage and the lateral hypothalamic syndrome. *J. Comp. Physiol. Psychol.* **87**, 808–830.

Mennini, T., Borroni, E., Samanin, R. and Garattini, S. (1981). Evidence of the existence of two different intraneuronal pools from which pharmacological agents can release serotonin. *Neurochem. Int.* (in press).

Neill, D. B. and Grossman, S. P. (1971). Interaction of the effects of reserpine and amphetamine on food and water intake. *J. Comp. Physiol. Psychol.* **76**, 327–336.

Nobin, A. and Björklund, A. (1978). Degenerative effects of various neurotoxic indoleamines on central monoamines neurons. *Ann. N.Y. Acad. Sci.* **305**, 305–327.

Offermeier, J. and du Preez, H. G. (1978). effects of anorectics on uptake and release of monoamines in synaptosomes. *In* "Central Mechanisms of Anorectic Drugs" (S. Garattini and R. Samanin, eds), pp. 217–231. Raven Press, New York.

Palkovitz, M., Brownstein, M., Saavedra, J. M. and Axelrod, J. (1974). Norepinephrine and dopamine content of hypothalamic nuclei of the rat. *Brain Res.* 77, 137–149.

Phillips, A. G. and Nikaido, R. S. (1975). Disruption of brain stimulation-induced feeding by dopamine receptor blockage. *Nature* 258, 750–751.

Pycock, C. J., Donaldson, I. M. and Marsden, C. D. (1975). Circling behaviour produced by unilateral lesions in the region of the locus coeruleus in rats. *Brain Res.* 97, 317–329.

Quattrone, A., Bendotti, C., Recchia, M. and Samanin, R. (1977). Various effects of d-amphetamine in rats with selective lesions of brain noradrenaline-containing neurons or treated with penfluridol. *Commun. Psychopharmac.* 1, 525–531.

Redmond, D. E. Jr, Huang, Y. H., Baulu, J., Snyder, D. R. and Maas, J. W. (1977). Norepinephrine and satiety in monkeys. *In* "Anorexia Nervosa" (R. A. Vigersky, ed.), pp. 81–96. Raven Press, New York.

Reid, W. D. (1970). Turnover rate of brain 5-hydroxytryptamine increased by d-amphetamine. *Brit. J. Pharmac.* 40, 483–491.

Robinson, R. G., McHugh, P. R. and Bloom, F. E. (1975b). Chlorpromazine induced hyperphagia in the rat. *Psychopharmac. Commun.* 1, 37–50.

Robinson, R. G., McHugh, P. R. and Folstein, M. F. (1975a). Measurement of appetite disturbances in psychiatric disorders. *J. Psychiatr. Res.* 12, 59–68.

Russek, M., Rodriguez-Zendejas, A. M. and Pina, S. (1968). Hypothetical liver receptors and the anorexia caused by adrenaline and glucose. *Physiol. Behav.* 3, 249–257.

Saller, C. F. and Stricker, E. M. (1976). Hyperphagia and increased growth in rats after intraventricular injection of 5, 7-dihydroxytryptamine. *Science* 192, 385–387.

Samanin, R., Bendotti, C., Bernasconi, S., Borroni, E. and Garattini, S. (1977b). Role of brain monoamines in the anorectic activity of mazindol and d-amphetamine in the rat. *Eur. J. Pharmac.* 43, 117–124.

Samanin, R., Bendotti, C., Bernasconi, S. and Pataccini, R. (1978). Differential role of brain monoamines in the activity of anorectic drugs. *In* "Central Mechanisms of Anorectic Drugs" (S. Garattini and R. Samanin, eds), pp. 233–242. Raven Press, New York.

Samanin, R., Bendotti, C., Miranda, F. and Garattini, S. (1977c). Decrease of food intake by quipazine in the rat: Relation to serotoninergic receptor stimulation. *J. Pharm. Pharmac.* 29, 53–54.

Samanin, R., Caccia, C., Bendotti, C., Borsini, F., Borroni, E., Invernizzi, R., Pataccini, R. and Mennini, T. (1980). Further studies on the mechanism of serotonin-dependent anorexia in rats. *Psychopharmacology* 68, 99–104.

Samanin, R., Ghezzi, D., Valzelli, L. and Garattini, S. (1972). The effects of selective lesioning of brain serotonin or catecholamine containing neurones on the anorectic activity of fenfluramine and amphetamine. *Eur. J. Pharmac.* 19, 318–322.

Samanin, R., Jori, A., Bernasconi, S., Morpurgo, E. and Garattini, S. (1977a). Biochemical and pharmacological studies on amineptine (S1694) and (+)-amphetamine in the rat. *J. Pharm. Pharmac.* 29, 555–558.

Samanin, R., Mennini, T., Ferraris, A., Bendotti, C., Borsini, F. and Garattini, S. (1979). m-Chlorophenylpiperazine; A central serotonin agonist causing powerful anorexia in rats. *Naunyn-Schmiedeberg's Arch. Pharmac.* 308, 159–163.

Schachter, S. (1968). Obesity and eating. *Science* 161, 751–756.

Schmitt, H. (1973). Influence d'agents interférant avec les catécholamines et la 5-hydroxytryptamine sur les effets anorexigènes de l'amphetamine et de la fenfluramine. *J. Pharmac.* (Paris) **4**, 285–294.

Schoot van der, J. B., Ariens, E. J., van Rossum, J. M. and Hurkmans, J. A. Th. (1962). Phenylisopropylamine derivatives, structure and action. *Arzneimittel-Forsch.* **12**, 902–907.

Silverstone, T. (1978). Psychopharmacology of anorectic drugs in man. Presented at C.I.N.P. International Congress, Vienna July 9–14.

Stunkard, A. J. (1955). The night-eating syndrome. A pattern of food intake among certain obese patients. *Amer. J. Med.* **19**, 78–85.

Valenstein, E. S. (1976). The interpetation of behavior evoked by brain stimulation. *In* "Brain-Stimulation Reward; (A. Wauquier and E. T. Rolls, eds), pp. 557–575. North Holland, Amsterdam.

Valenstein, E. S. (1977). Brain mechanisms of reinforcement. *In* "Neurosurgical Treatment to Psychiatry, Pain and Epilepsy" (W. H. Sweet, S. Obrador and J. G. Martin-Rodriguez, eds), pp. 27–50. University Park Press, Baltimore.

Van Rossum, J. M. Schoot van der, J. B. and Hurkmans, J. A. Th. (1962). Mechanism of action of cocaine and amphetamine in the brain. *Experientia* **18**, 229–231.

Wise, R. A., Spindler, J., De Wit, H. and Gerber, G. J. (1978). Neuroleptic-induced "anhedonia" in rats: pimozide blocks reward quality of food. *Science* **201**, 262–264.

Wurtman, J. J. and Wurtman, R. J. (1977). Fenfluramine and fluoxetine spare protein consumption while suppressing caloric intake by rats. *Science* **198**, 1178–1180.

Wurtman, J. J. and Wurtman, R. J. (1979). Drugs that enhance central serotoninergic transmission diminish elective carbohydrate consumption by rats. *Life Sci.* **24**, 895–904.

Yokel, R. A. and Wise, R. A. (1976). Attenuation of intravenous amphetamine reinforcement by central dopamine blockade in rats. *Psychopharmacology* **48**, 311–318.

Zinace, R. J. and Rutledge, C. O. (1972). A comparison of the effects of fenfluramine and amphetamine on uptake, release and catabolism of norepinephrine in rat brain. *J. Pharmac. exp. Ther.* **180**, 118–126.

# 3 ☐ Behavioural Pharmacology of Feeding

J. E. Blundell and C. J. Latham

## I. BASIC STRATEGIES

The term behavioural pharmacology represents a coalition between two scientific disciplines, psychology and pharmacology. In general, the term can refer to any instance in which some aspect of behaviour is monitored in conjunction with a pharmacological manipulation, and in the study of feeding, the most frequently chosen behavioural variable has been the weight of food consumed. However, the complexities of behaviour far exceed such a simple dependent variable, and the development of the field of behavioural pharmacology of feeding will depend upon the establishment of a set of sophisticated procedures for the analysis of feeding behaviour. This set of procedures will complement the elegance and precision of chemical and biological techniques used in the design of drugs and in the analysis of their effects upon neurochemical and physiological systems. There are clear signs that experimental psychologists and other scientists can provide the refinement of behavioural conceptualization required to expand the study of the behavioural pharmacology of feeding.

This field of study embraces research both in applied and pure science, and incorporates three major purposes (e.g. Thompson and Schuster, 1968). First, behavioural pharmacology has grown along with the increasing interest of pharmaceutical companies in the development of anti-obesity drugs. This enterprise has needed testing procedures to determine which of the thousands of new compounds produced by pharmaceutical chemists display clinically desirable behavioural activity. In turn, this undertaking is dominated by pragmatic considerations, and there are obvious practical reasons why any potential compound can receive only limited attention. Accordingly, the "screening" problem has promoted the development of quick and simple procedures for the rapid classification of many compounds, and for the evaluation of their potential usefulness in clinical practice. A second purpose of behavioural pharmacology involves the use of detailed behavioural procedures for the investigation of the mechanisms of drug action. When subjected to refined analysis, many categories of behaviour reveal a complex structure within which adjustments may occur at many points without necessarily being accompanied by crude shifts in the "total quantity of behaviour". This is true of food consumption, and changes in subtle features of the pattern of feeding behaviour may be used to throw light upon the mode of action of the drug causing the change.

A third and major purpose of behavioural pharmacology of feeding is the use of drugs as tools to explore the structure of complex behaviour or to investigate the relationship between physiological happenings and behavioural events. In this way, drugs can be used as pharmacological scalpels to dissect the components of natural systems governing food consumption and the regulation of body weight in order to reveal the properties of these systems. In certain circumstances, drugs can show how biological systems function. To achieve this purpose, the behavioural pharmacology of feeding must be concerned as much with overeating (hyperphagia) as with undereating (hypophagia) and must devote as much attention to the qualitative aspects of feeding as it does to quantitative features. This chapter mainly will be concerned with these two last purposes of behavioural pharmacology: the use of behavioural analysis as a tool to understand the action of a drug, and the use of drugs as tools to understand the workings of bio-behavioural systems.

## II. MANIPULATIONS OF THE FEEDING SYSTEM

Is body weight regulated? Is food intake controlled in the interests of this regulation? The natural answer to both of these questions is "yes", based on what Waddington (1977) would refer to as the "conventional wisdom of the dominant group". However, some recent discussions of these issues have suggested that the answers are not quite so obvious. It is noticeable that for many animals, including man, once the period of rapid growth has occurred, the body size remains fairly constant over long periods of time. This observation has led some theorists to suppose that the size of the body, or some feature correlated with body size, is actively regulated. The notion of regulation is consistent with the principle of homeostasis which is extensively applied to biological functioning and which has led to the search for mechanisms responsible for the regulation of various bodily parameters (e.g. Yamamoto and Brobeck, 1965). One suggestion is that biological constancy in body weight is maintained by reference to a "set point" embodied in physiological mechanisms which in turn control energy intake and expenditure (e.g. Keesey, 1978; Mrosovsky and Powley, 1977). Other theorists have argued that features such as total body energy, body fat or body weight are not actively regulated about prescribed set values but that apparent constancy is maintained by a natural balance between intake and output (Booth, 1976; Garrow, 1978).

Moreover, it is known that stability within a controlled system can be maintained by a regulatory system which does not contain a set point; the term "settling point" may give a more appropriate description of the working of such a system (Wirtshafter and Davis, 1977; Davis and Wirtshafter, 1978).

Indeed, it has been argued that, "in the absence of physiological identification of a comparator device, it is unnecessary to assume that a regulatory homeostatic system contains such a mechanism. The term "set point" may be valuable as a conceptual convenience, provided it is realized that it does not imply a physiological or structural entity" (Wolff, 1976 p. 227).

This debate focusses on two issues: whether or not there is active regulation of body weight, and whether this regulation requires the involvement of a set-point mechanism. The view taken by the present authors is that we are dealing with a system which displays regulatory or stabilizing properties but which does not necessitate the existence of a set-point device. Such a system would appear to operate by attempting to match food intake to nutritional requirements and energy expenditure, and it seems likely that the system has evolved to achieve this result. It is of course recognized that certain processes involved in this matching will operate in anticipation of future events rather than as mere reflex responses to an induced change. Indeed, since one of the most threatening circumstances for an organism is the scarcity of nutrients and physical deficit, it may be surmised that anticipatory processes to confer protection against such a possibility would be favoured through natural selection. In other words, a defensive strategy would be to err towards over-consumption, a feature which may account, in part, for the vulnerability of some animals (including man) to develop obesity.

This discussion is not trite, for it is important to establish that feeding behaviour is not an arbitrary activity but belongs to a rational system incorporating purposive capacity. Moreover, critical processes in this system (Fig. 1) can be identified. Since food consumption can be disturbed, temporarily at least, by a vast variety of influences, when discussing pharmacological manipulations it will be necessary to establish that the behavioural adjustment has been achieved through intervention in the system which operates to match intake to requirements rather than via some non-specific interference. This is particularly important when drugs are used as tools to explore the mechanisms of the bio-behavioural system.

The stabilization of body weight and the maintenance of bodily constituents at preferred values depends on a complex physiological system in which metabolic, neural and hormonal signals are integrated into a coherent pattern as considered in Chapter 1. The basic elements of such a system are set out in Fig. 1 which illustrates the inter-relationship between behavioural and physiological processes. The system shows how post-ingestional signals together with metabolic signals arising from the processing of nutrients, may be brought together to provide the basis of a link between central and peripheral mechanisms. It follows that shifts in food consumption or in the stabilized level of body weight may be brought about by alterations occurring at many points in this network. In turn, therapeutic techniques, for example in obesity, may be directed at these sites of disregulation (Blundell and Rogers, 1978). Hunger may be controlled by psycho-therapeutic or behavioural strategies directed at point A. The process of eating (point B) may be constrained in a mild way by adherence to calorie-controlled diets or more severely, by enforced starvation

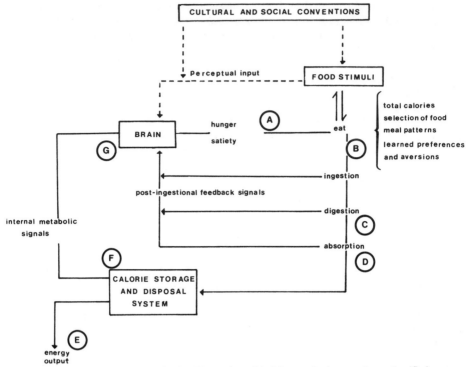

*Fig. 1.* Working conceptualization illustrating critical features in the complex and unified system influencing feeding (see text for explanation).

in a metabolic ward or jaw-clamping by means of a dental splint. The process of digestion may be directly inhibited by gastroplasty which effectively reduces the volume of the stomach (point C) while absorption of nutrients can be obstructed by the ileojejunum by-pass operation (point D). In turn, the basic metabolic rate or energy output may be increased by a regime of physical exercise (point E) and there are instances of cosmetic surgery being carried out to remove adipose tissue directly (point F). More dramatically, brain surgery (point G) has been performed in an attempt to destroy central mechanisms responsible for hunger motivation.

Two important points arise from this consideration of obesity treatments. First, eating is a resilient activity which resists attempts to suppress it. In those circumstances in which the purpose has been to directly block eating, the behaviour is resumed with equal or greater intensity once the blockade is removed. Secondly, interventions which appear to deal with portions of the system not directly related to eating have repercussions upon the amount of food taken in. It is of course well known that physical exercise will lead to increased consumption (e.g. James, 1980). Less obvious is the finding that a reduction in food intake is one major consequence of the removal of a portion of the absorptive intestine. This has been shown to occur in animals (Sclafani *et al.*, 1978) and in man (e.g. Mills and Stunkard, 1976) and it has been calculated that reduced intake accounts for about three quarters of the total caloric deficit observed following surgery (Bray, 1978). These findings indicate that feeding behaviour can be altered, often in a counter-intuitive manner, by procedures not primarily directed towards the control of intake. The system operates as a cohesive unit and perturbations in one domain will set up vibrations which will be felt elsewhere.

It follows that adjustments in feeding behaviour can arise from pharmacological manipulations at many points in the feeding system and consequently, the interpretation of the effects of drugs on food intake is often not straightforward. For example, eating may be altered by drugs which act directly to inhibit or enhance hunger or satiety (point A). In addition, drugs acting on digestive activities or modifying the physico-chemical characteristics of the stomach (point C) may alter the processing of ingested nutrients and may have repercussions upon the act of eating itself. The compound ($\pm$)-transexpoxyaconitic acid is known to slow the rate of gastric emptying and to reduce food consumption in rats. In addition, inhibitors of pancreatic $\alpha$-amylase can effectively reduce the bio-availability of carbohydrate by preventing the digestion of starch to maltose and consequently diminishing the amount of glucose available for absorption. Moreover, various pharmacological agents interfere with nutrient absorption in other ways. Neomycin and cholestyramine partially obstruct the absorption of fat, and perfluoroctyl bromide reduces general nutrient absorption by providing an inert film of material over the stomach and intestines.

By analogy with the results of intestinal by-pass surgery, it may be expected that any interference with intestinal function will bring about secondary changes in food intake. Among those compounds which are known to modify lipid synthesis (point F), the most thoroughly researched is ($-$)-hydroxycitrate (Sullivan *et al.*, 1974). In rats, this agent has been shown to reduce circulating levels of triglycerides and to reduce body weight (Sullivan *et al.*, 1977). It also exerts a marked effect on food intake. Considerable attention is currently being devoted to the family of agents known as thermogenic drugs which, as the term implies, serve to divert calories into heat production and ultimately heat loss from the body. It is clear that thermogenesis is an important factor in energy balance (Rothwell and Stock, 1979) and since increases or decreases in food consumption lead to compensatory adjustments in heat production, it can be expected that facilitation or inhibition of thermogenesis will result in corresponding changes in food intake in order to maintain the balance of energy in the body.

Many of the pharmacological procedures discussed above have come into prominence through the research effort directed to the development of antiobesity compounds (see Sullivan, 1979, for review). However, with regard to the behavioural pharmacology of feeding, the important theoretical principle to emerge is that various aspects of food consumption can be modified by drugs acting at a variety of sites in the body. This issue should be kept in mind particularly when drugs are used as tools to investigate the mechanisms underlying adjustments in feeding behaviour.

## III.  THE BIO-PYSCHOLOGICAL VIEW

### A.  Interactionist Position

The preceding discussion has dealt with ways in which changes in food consumption can arise through interactions at a variety of sites in the internal environment. Indeed, since transient change in eating can be brought about by a multitude of factors, the problem is how to distinguish non-specific interference from specific modulation of the physiological system. In addition, it is abundantly clear that feeding activities are strongly influenced by changes going on outside the animal: in its external environment. Consequently, feeding behaviour can only be properly understood as an interaction between two domains: a world of events conducted under the skin and a world of happenings beyond the skin. Figure 2 lists some of the important features of the external environment. Naturally, many of these are concerned with the nature of the food supply including its flavour, texture, composition and variety. Changes in these parameters alone are often sufficient to induce large shifts in food consumption and in body weight.

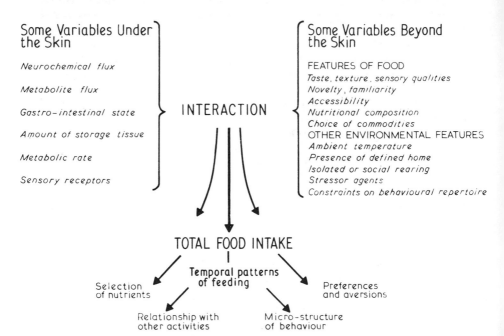

*Fig. 2.*  Feeding viewed as an interaction between two domains of events.

In addition to factors association with food *per se*, a diverse range of other environmental variables can modify short-term or long-term food consumption. These variables include the prevailing environmental temperature, the presence of other animals, and various physical aspects of the environment including cage size, presence of a definite home compartment and those structural qualities which limit the mobility of the animal and its ability to fulfil a range of activities in its behavioural repertoire. Ultimately, the behaviour displayed by any animal will result from interplay between events under the skin and those existing beyond the skin.

## B. The Structure of Behaviour

In many studies on the effects of drugs on brain function and feeding, it is noticeable that the techniques for measuring neural parameters are more sophisticated than those for measuring food consumption. Delicate and sensitive procedures are often employed to reveal the effects of drugs on selected neurochemical events in particular brain zones, thus providing a detailed picture of the effects of pharmacological intervention under the skin. On the other hand, feeding is often measured by simply measuring the weight of food taken from a dish or hopper over a brief period of time. In many instances, an animal may be deprived of food for a given period before being exposed to the pharmacological procedure intended to adjust caloric intake.

However, it can be demonstrated that mammalian food intake comprises complex behaviour sequences and constitutes a discontinuous process in which periods of eating alternate with periods of non-eating. Freely-feeding animals eat in discrete meals (Richter, 1927) and within meals, short bouts of eating are separated by short episodes of other behavioural activities (e.g. Wiepkema, 1971a). Accordingly, it is possible to measure feeding by assessing various parameters of meal patterns such as the number of meals taken over a given period, meal sizes, meal durations, inter-meal intervals and certain relationships between these variables such as the ratio of meal size to pre- or post-meal interval (e.g. Le Magnen and Tallon, 1968). In addition, certain intra-meal characteristics may be assessed, such as the number, size and duration of eating bouts and the relationship between bouts of eating and non-eating activities (Wiepkema, 1971b). These techniques draw attention to the distinction between food intake (usually assessed by measuring the weight of food consumed) and feeding behaviour which can only be understood through a close analysis of the topography of the eating response. Although measurement of the sheer bulk of food consumed may throw light upon certain features of energy balance, it seems likely that a more detailed behavioural analysis will be required to determine the way in which brain processes exert a moment to moment control over feeding activities.

In order to capitalize fully on a behavioural analysis, it will be necessary to provide the animal with the opportunity to display a full range of behaviours in the feeding repertoire. In many experiments, the repertoire is artificially restricted by allowing access to a single food for a limited period of time and subjecting the animal to severe deprivation which enforces rapid and often frantic eating. It has been proposed that only those studies of eating behaviour in freely-feeding animals provide data to illustrate how an animal is matched to its ecological niche (Collier *et al.*, 1972). In addition, Fig. 2 shows how the artificial restriction of an animal's environment will contaminate the inter-action between the biological and behavioural domains. It follows that the operations of the interacting process can be most thoroughly understood by allowing the opportunity for a fairly free expression of behaviour and by measuring not only the total caloric intake but also monitoring patterns of feeding, the selection of particular nutrients and the occurrence of particular preferences for highly preferred commodities and aversions for undesirable foods.

## C. Motivation and Behaviour

The experimental environment within which feeding is measured is import-ant, for the data are frequently used to establish that changes in consumption have been brought about by alterations in presumed motives such as hunger or appetite. There are certain conceptual difficulties surrounding the use of these terms (see Blundell, 1980, for discussion) but they most commonly refer to an animal's tendency to seek food purposively and its willingness to initiate consumption. It is tempting for researchers to ascribe any changes in food intake to a modification of either hunger or appetite. However, in the study of motivational states in animals, certain principles have been informally estab-lished for the evaluation of motivation. Generally speaking, animals must display an expenditure of effort or a toleration of aversive stimulation in pursuit of the goal objects. The classical study is the investigation of motiva-tion in rats with lesions of the ventro-medial hypothalamus (Miller *et al.*, 1950) which demonstrates that these animals consume more food than their un-lesioned counterparts, but perform less well on all tests of motivation, at least during the static phase of their obesity. Thus before the labels hunger and appetite can properly be assigned to changes in feeding, the data must include much more information than the mere crude weight of food consumed (Miller, 1955).

An examination of the structure of feeding activities reveals a highly orga-nized sequence of actions which have a clearly defined beginning and end. It should be noted at the outset, that there is a strong possibility that mechanisms responsible for the *initiation* of an episode of feeding may differ from the mechanisms which *maintain* the behaviour (see also Chapter 1). Considering the physiological mechanisms controlling maternal behaviour (an activity with a topography similar to feeding) Lamb (1975) has suggested that the balance of hormones influence the motivated aspects of the behaviour, whereas limbic system structures are responsible for the integration and organization of the sequence of acts. This distinction mirrors the separation of *appetitive* and *consummatory* phases of behaviour. It is clear that if drugs are to be used to explore the mechanisms influencing food intake, it will be necessary to distinguish changes in motivation from changes in integration, both of which may produce similar effects on the total amount of food eaten.

## D. Conceptual Ability

An interactional view of feeding (Fig. 2) may suggest the idea that behaviour results from a collision between internal and external forces, with behaviour being dominated by the strongest force arising out of the fragments of the collision. However, the interaction between internal and external events can be better understood as a rational relationship. Nothing is more important to animals than that they approach and consume foods which are beneficial and avoid foods which are harmful. It is now known that powerful and sensitive processes exist to allow animals to acquire knowledge about their nutritional environment (e.g. Garcia *et al.* 1975; Rozin, 1976) and to adapt their behaviour in an appropriate way. In response to various demands for the procurement and consumption of food, animals will modify their pattern of behaviour to maintain a level of intake compatible with other behavioural requirements (Collier, 1977). To the naïve observer, it often appears as if animals blindly scurry about their environments responding with reflex actions to various stimuli. Yet animals do have conceptual capacities, and they develop understanding of the conditions in which they exist. Although laboratory animals appear to have time to spare, spending much of their days resting and relaxing, it is worth considering that all organisms have obligations to fulfil and commitments to meet; bio-psychological imperatives govern the behavioural repertoires of rats just as they govern our own.

Of course the conceptual ability of man far exceeds that of a rat and involves qualitatively different processes, but observations and experiments have shown that rats possess considerable adaptive strategies. Since there are no *in vitro* models of behaviour, it is often tempting for researchers to regard animals in cages as living test-tubes, providing a simple and objective behavioural assay. We feel that some bodies of data would be better understood if it was recognized that animals act in a rational manner to protect and conserve themselves, and often display anticipatory behaviour in the interests of bio-logical harmony. A bio-psychological view of feeding encourages consideration of an interaction between the biological and psychological domains, draws attention to the structure of behaviour and its motivational properties, and acknowledges the conceptual ability of all organisms. When drugs are administered to animals, they intervene in a complex and sophisticated matrix of interwoven systems.

## IV. SOME METHODOLOGICAL ISSUES IN THE MEASUREMENT OF FEEDING

A good deal of work in the behavioural pharmacology of feeding has been prompted by the research and development of anti-obesity drugs. Since the pharmaceutical industry requires screening procedures for new compounds that can be administered rapidly and simply, one common technique for the measurement of feeding consists of weighing the amount of food consumed by animals (usually rats) using a discrete test interval (usually 1 or 2 h) following a period of food deprivation (e.g. Tedeschi, 1966). Alternatively, animals may be placed on cyclic training programmes when they are obliged to eat at specific times during the day when allowed access to food. These techniques have been widely used since anti-obesity drugs are developed as a commercial exercise rather than for the convenience of theoretical biology. However, there are reasons for believing that such simple procedures, derived from screening tests, are not effective either for producing precise information about drug action or for throwing light upon the processes controlling feeding behaviour.

First, a simple measure of the weight of food consumed in a discrete interval of time may conceal information about the manner in which a drug has adjusted consumption. For example, an animal may fail to eat because of the non-specific disruption of any controlled sequential behaviour by competing or interfering activities. Indeed it now seems likely that a large part of the inhibitory action of high doses of (+)-amphetamine on food intake can be accounted for by the inability of animals to eat due to stereotypy or excessive hyperactivity. On the other hand, animals may be induced to overeat due to heightened arousal (Jacobs and Farel, 1968) or to some other effect of stressor agents (Robbins and Fray, 1980). In either of these circumstances, a single measure of weight of food consumed fails to indicate whether a drug is acting to adjust the onset of eating, to slow or speed up the rate of eating, or to influence the termination of an eating episode.

Secondly, although brief periods of eating following long periods of deprivation are typical for drug experiments, they are not typical of animal behaviour and are not usually encountered in natural animal feeding repertoires. Consequently, it is possible that drugs are being evaluated under highly abnormal circumstances (Collier et al., 1972; Hirsch and Collier, 1974; Moran, 1975). Thirdly, it is known that food deprivation can modify brain neurotransmitter systems (Curzon et al., 1972; Perez-Cruet et al., 1972). Since many drugs, particularly certain anti-obesity compounds, are believed to exert their action via central neurochemical processes it follows that drugs administered to severely deprived animals may be intervening in atypical brain metabolism.

The most critical issue concerns the question of food deprivation which, contrary to general belief, may present a methodological barrier to further understanding of the effect of drugs on feeding. To illustrate this question, it is worth inquiring what period of food restriction in man would be required to produce a level of deprivation equivalent to the withholding of food for 24 h in the rat (intervals of 20–24 h are commonly encountered in animal studies). When this question was posed at a recent international conference, the replies ranged from 3 to 5 days. Accordingly, it may be questioned whether the observation of human eating following such lengthy episodes would cast much light on human feeding mechanisms, and whether such a technique should be adopted as the standard procedure for drug testing in man.

In summary, the techniques which have defined the orthodox approach to the measurement of feeding in animals for many years may possess inherent deficiencies which hinder their usefulness. The combined use of severe deprivation periods and short food tests represent a procedure which may be highly insensitive to certain drug effects: masking the action of a weak acting drug and grossly exaggerating the effect of a powerful drug (Latham and Blundell, 1979). In addition, this procedure may create circumstances for the appearance of abnormal behaviour and may modify drug action in an unknown way by altering brain chemistry. It seems appropriate now for investigations in the behavioural pharmacology of feeding to develop within a framework of bio-psychological principles.

## V. DEVELOPMENTS IN THE ANALYSIS OF FEEDING BEHAVIOUR

The short history of the behavioural pharmacology of feeding reveals a preoccupation with measurement of the effects of drugs in deprived animals given brief feeding tests with standard laboratory foods. Deprivation has been the major independent variable used to engender changes in the potentiality to feed, while the weight of laboratory chow consumed represents the primary dependent variable. These conditions fail to sample adequately the varied circumstances which influence feeding behaviour, and it should be appreciated that certain deductions concerning the mechanisms of drug action are based on information from only a limited fragment of an animal's feeding repertoire. The behavioural pharmacology of feeding would certainly be enriched and strengthened by the gathering of more detailed evidence about the qualitative features of feeding behaviour together with a consideration of meaningful circumstances, in addition to food restriction, which promote changes in an animal's tendency to feed.

The impetus given to the pharmacology of feeding by the interest in anti-obesity agents has ensured that considerable attention has been directed to ways of inducing animals to overeat. The genetically fat mouse (ob/ob) and rat (fa/fa), both of which display hyperphagia leading to obesity, have been employed, but more enthusiasm has been directed to the phenomenon of obesity induced by brain treatments. Of particular importance for this approach have been the baso-medial portion of the hypothalamus and certain well-defined neurotransmitter pathways such as the ventral noradrenergic bundle. For example, a number of anorexic drugs including amphetamine, phenmetrazine and chlorphentermine were tested for their effectiveness in mice made hyperphagic and obese by treatment with aurothiogucose (Friedman et al., 1962). In general, these drugs produced a greater suppression of food intake in the obese animals. Similar effects have been reported with amphetamine in animals which have been made hyperphagic by electrolytic or radio-frequency lesions of the medial hypothalamus (e.g. Epstein, 1959; Reynolds, 1959). Fenfluramine also appears to exert a stronger effect in lesioned animals than in controls

(Bernier *et al.*, 1969). However, owing to the widespread behavioural and physiological perturbations brought about by hypothalamic lesions, the interpretation of drug effects in these studies is far from clear. Indeed, understanding of the behavioural actions of anorexic drugs may be enhanced if feeding behaviour were measured in animals which had not been subjected to severe brain damage.

## A.  Dietary Induced Hyperphagia

Although brain treatments provided an alternative to food deprivation for the promotion of eating in experimental animals, the studies have generally employed deprivation periods and standard laboratory food for the actual measurement of drug effects. For these reasons, the studies should be considered in the light of the criticisms set out in the previous section. In addition, although it has been strongly implied that obesity induced by brain treatments in animals provides a reasonable model for human obesity (Schachter, 1971; Mrosovsky, 1971), the evidence is equivocal. In recent years, greater attention has been given to the idea that environmental factors, particularly those related to diet, may play a role in the development of obesity. Certainly, dietary manipulations can alter an animal's tendency to eat, and it seems appropriate that the behavioural pharmacology of feeding should now expand to investigate drug effects on feeding in the presence of foodstuffs different from the balanced diet of laboratory chow.

The literature on dietary-induced overeating and dietary obesity has recently been reviewed by Kanarek and Hirsch (1977) and Sclafani (1978), and in both cases emphasis has been given to three particular conditions. First, it has been known since the early experiments of Ingle (1949) that rats and mice display marked increases in body weight when presented with a high fat diet. In general, rats prefer greasy diets to dry laboratory chow and display hyperphagia (Hamilton, 1964). However, the overeating is reflected in the total calories consumed rather than the weight of food eaten. Indeed, rats may reduce the amount of food taken in, but consume a surplus of calories owing to the caloric density of the fatty food. In addition, obesity may be promoted by an increased efficiency in the deposition of fatty foods into adipose tissue (Schemmel, Mickelson and Tolgay, 1969).

Secondly, rats can be persuaded to overeat and to develop mild obesity by increasing the carbohydrate content of diets. This can be achieved by directly adding in a high-carbohydrate substance like sucrose to a standard diet or, more effectively, by offering animals separate access to a sucrose solution in addition to the normal diet (Kanarek and Hirsch, 1977). When young rats were provided with a laboratory food together with a 32% sucrose solution small increases in daily calorie intake were observed, but these were not translated into additional weight gain until the animals were about 70 days old. Accordingly, age is an important variable influencing this phenomenon as is the type of carbohydrate used as the supplement.

The third and most celebrated form of dietary obesity involves the induction of overeating and weight gain by giving animals access to a variety of highly palatable commodities including cheese, bread, biscuits, chocolate, salami and sausages. This powerful procedure was given substance and credibility by Sclafani and Springer (1976) who charted the phenomenon and outlined its major features. This form of dietary-induced hyperphagia depends on the use of a snack-food diet, and has recently been taken up by a number of researchers who have referred to the dietary manipulations as cafeteria feeding, the super-market diet, varied diets or palatable diets. An example of this phenomenon is illustrated in Fig. 3 which shows that the addition of just two extra foods, say bread and chocolate, to laboratory chow can lead to a dramatic increase in energy intake and to almost a doubling of the body weight of female rats over a period of some 5 months (Rogers and Blundell, 1980). This figure also demon-strates that the hyperphagia was brought about initially by an increase in both the number and the size of meals. However, during the development of the obesity, meal frequency declined so that eventually the increase in meal size became totally responsible for the hyperphagia. These changes have been interpreted as indicating the separate contribution of *variety* and *palatability* to the development of dietary-induced hyperphagia.

It is clear that these procedures exploit a portion of the feeding repertoire which is not embraced by studies involving food deprivation and laboratory chow. Accordingly, they permit a wider sampling of the range of variables known to influence feeding. An analysis of the effects of pharmacological manipulation on dietary-induced hyperphagia would considerably extend the theoretical base for understanding drug-feeding interactions.

## B. Appetite and Hedonism: Dietary Hyperphagia and Drug Hypotheses

Considering the motivational aspects of eating in animals it has been argued that a distinction can be made between the effects of hunger and appetite (Sclafani and Kluge, 1974; Blundell, 1980). Hunger is generated by a deficit signal and primarily influences the onset of eating, whereas appetite is engen-dered by certain qualitative features of the diet and exerts a primary control over the maintenance of eating (but see Introduction and Chapter 1 for alternative views). According to our usage of the term, appetite is modulated by textural and taste characteristics of food. Accordingly, the increases in eating brought about by high-fat diets which alter the texture of the food, by carbohydrate diets which adjust the taste, or by snack-food diets which modify taste and texture can be regarded as predominantly due to increase in appetite. It follows that these techniques provide a means of examining the effect of pharmacological agents on hunger or appetite. Manipulations which lead to a more severe adjustment in snack-food eating than in the eating of laboratory chow can be inferred to exert a potent effect on appetite. On the other hand, drugs which bring about an equal suppression (or enhancement) of deprivation-induced eating of snack foods or chow may be regarded as displaying a primary effect on hunger.

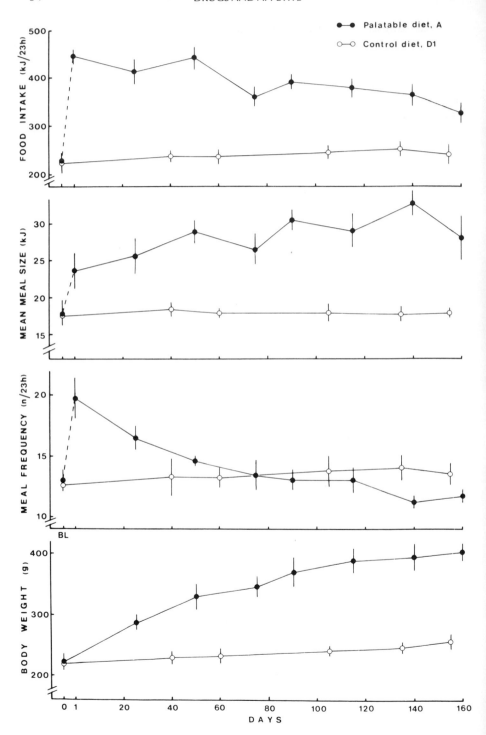

*Fig. 3.* Long-term changes in food intake, body weight, meal size and meal frequency brought about by offering female rats a varied and palatable diet.

At the present time, very few pharmacological manipulations of dietary hyperphagia have been reported. Some years ago, Roszkowski and Kelley (1963) tested the effect of certain anorexic drugs in a brief feeding test during which rats were offered a highly preferred beef broth. Amphetamine, phenmetrazine, diethylpropion, phendimetrazine and a number of experimental compounds markedly suppressed the consumption of broth. However, the potency of the drugs in this situation was not compared with their potency to suppress intake of less preferred foods. Although the authors regarded their test as a measure of

> . . . appetite as distinct from hunger. This should not be construed to indicate a selective suppression of appetite rather than hunger; in all probability the drugs studied indiscriminantly suppress all feeding behaviour (p. 372).

It is clear that in order to distinguish between effects on hunger and appetite, the experimental procedure must embody a comparison of the potency of drugs to inhibit eating of highly preferred and less preferred foods.

More recently, one study has reported the effect of the anti-obesity drug fenfluramine in suppressing the hyperphagia and obesity induced by continual access to a snack-food diet comprising various types of biscuits, fruit, chocolate and sugar-coated cereals. The drug was administered in the drinking water to provide a daily dosage of approximately 10 mg/kg. This treatment effectively blocked the rapid rise in body weight induced by the supermarket diet. This study certainly indicates the power of an anti-obesity agent to inhibit dietary-induced obesity but since no comparison groups were included, it is not possible to deduce the mechanisms responsible for the effect (Kirby et al., 1978).

If it is regarded that appetite reflects the hedonic value of food, the perceived pleasantness of the sensory qualities (taste, texture, etc.) of the diet, then pharmacological manipulations believed to adjust brain mechanisms mediating the hedonic response would be expected to markedly suppress appetite. Expressed operationally, these agents should exert a comparatively greater effect on dietary hyperphagia than on the consumption of a bland food. Three possibilities are worth considering. First, arising from the postulated role for dopamine systems in brain-reward processes (e.g. German and Bowden, 1974; Wise, 1978) it has been suggested that neuroleptic drugs (dopamine receptor blockers), which generally reduce the rate of responding for rewarding brain stimulation, may bring about "anhedonia". It has been reported that the neuroleptic pimozide attenuates lever-pressing and running for food reward in hungry rats (Wise et al., 1978). This finding led to the suggestion that "pimozide appears to selectively blunt the rewarding impact of food and other hedonic stimuli" (p. 262). One implication is that pimozide, together with other neuroleptic drugs, exerts a primary effect on appetite rather than hunger, at least in animal studies. Since pimozide fails to block the onset of eating episodes (Blundell et al., 1977), any effect of pimozide on hunger is likely to be slight, and since pimozide slows the rate of eating (Blundell and Latham, 1978) this is further suggestive evidence that the major action is via appetite. Moreover, if the net hedonic value of a snack food diet is greater than that of laboratory chow, then it follows that pimozide should exert a powerful selective effect on dietary-induced hyperphagia through its effect on appetite.

A secondary issue concerns the postulated role for the endogenous opiates or endorphins in behaviour. As Goldstein (1976) pointed out, it is probably misleading to think of opiate receptors as exclusively mediating analgesia, and one could suppose that "endorphins play some central role in the control of affective states and possibly also of appetitive drives (food, water, sex) known to be associated with limbic system functioning" (p. 1085). On the basis of certain limited studies with genetically obese rats and mice (Margules *et al.*, 1978), it has been suggested that excess pituitary $\beta$-endorphin may play a role in the hyperphagia and development of obesity. Although certain of these findings have been disputed (Rossier *et al.*, 1979), the proposed function of endorphins in certain aspects of pleasure and reward (Belluzi and Stein, 1977) suggests that endogenous neuropeptides may be involved in the mediation of the satisfaction derived from eating. In other words, it can be proposed that endorphins influence eating through appetite but not hunger. If this is the case, then manipulation of the endorphin system should lead to marked changes in snack-food eating. It is known that the opiate antagonist naloxone can attenuate feeding (Holtzman, 1974) and it can be hypothesized that this antagonist would exert a pronounced suppression of dietary-induced hyperphagia.

Thirdly, dietary overeating can be considered in relation to the proposed role for serotonin in feeding (Blundell, 1977, 1978). Evidence suggests that this neurotransmitter may be involved in mediating the process of satiation and the state of satiety. It is clear that the processes of appetite and satiation are reciprocally related. As satiation is intensified, so appetite diminishes (see Blundell, 1980). Consequently pharmacological manipulations which promote the process of satiation will automatically lead to a suppression of appetite at some stage during feeding episodes. It follows that drugs which bring about activation of serotonin systems may be expected to decrease appetite whereas drugs which block serotonin receptors or slow the rate of release or synthesis should enhance appetite. These hypotheses can be tested readily by comparing the effectiveness of these agents to adjust the eating of palatable and bland foods.

There is no doubt that a number of other hypotheses could be developed to establish the relationship between drugs and the hyperphagic response to palatability and variety. It is to be hoped that researchers will make increasing use of dietary-induced overeating to broaden understanding of the action of drugs on wider aspects of the feeding repertoires of animals.

## C. Arousal-induced Eating

The idea that feeding can be instigated by various states of arousal unrelated to either the nutritional state of an organism or to characteristics of food is both controversial and important. The significance of this issue rests on its power to substantiate one frequently mooted cause of human obesity. It is often assumed that humans eat in response to anxiety, stress or to various emotional variables. In turn, the psychosomatic view postulates that the act of eating represents a coping strategy which acquires reward value through the termination of an aversive state. Although this view is widely held, it is not supported by any firm body of evidence but rather by the strength of clinical judgements and intuitive assertions. Hence, in this form, the notion of stress-induced eating is controversial.

Recently, this domain of research has been reviewed by Robbins and Fray (1980) who concluded that the phenomena of arousal-induced eating is a clearly established fact, though it does not invariably occur in either animals or man. These authors favour the explanation that organisms (including man) respond to activation by focussing on salient external cues. The eating behaviour is then maintained by its own reinforcing consequences and results in metabolic changes which generate the internal changes associated with eating. In this way, it is argued, the state induced by activation or stress may come to be virtually indistinguishable from natural hunger.

Widespread commitment to the role of emotionalty and stress in human overeating together with new explanations for its mechanism, suggest a need to develop an animal model which can be used to examine the effects of pharmacological manipulation. It has been proposed that eating induced by electrical stimulation of the lateral hypothalamus represents a form of non-specific activation induced eating (Valenstien *et al.*, 1970). In turn, it has been reported that an anorexic agent like amphetamine antagonizes lateral hypothalamic-induced eating (Stark and Totty, 1967; Thode and Carlisle, 1968). Recently, a more convincing model of stress-induced eating has been developed (Antelman and Szechtman, 1975; Antelman *et al.*, 1975). It has been shown that a mild non-specific stress brought about by applying constant pressure to a rat's tail by means of a haemostat can reliably induce eating in sated rats. The behaviour occurs with a short latency, appears quite normal and apparently proceeds without obvious pain. Moreover, when the "tail-pinch" was applied several times daily, rats overate on a highly preferred food and markedly increased body weight (Rowland and Antelman, 1976).

There is now a considerable body of data on the pharmacology of tail-pinch-induced eating, almost all of which has been collected by Antelman and his colleagues. First, the initial observation that tail-pinch produced gnawing and licking suggested that the pharmacological analysis could profitably follow guidelines previously established for the examination of amphetamine-induced stereotypy. It was immediately discovered that the dopamine receptor blockers haloperidol, spiroperidol and pimozide brought about a marked attenuation of tail-pinch-induced eating. In contrast, adrenergic blocking agents such as phentolamine, phenoxybenzamine, propranolol and sotalol had no effect. Interestingly, the atypical neuroleptics clozapine and thioridazine failed to attenuate tail-pinch eating, a finding which is paralleled by the failure of these agents to attenuate amphetamine anorexia (Burridge and Blundell, 1979). In keeping with the observed effects of typical neuroleptics, $\alpha$-methyl-p-tyrosine blocked tail-pinch eating while FLA-63 did not. These data suggested that the induced eating depended on newly synthesized dopamine. Since lesioning of the nigro-striatal pathways by means of the neurotoxin 6-OHDA injected directly into the $A_9$ region produced a significant deficit in the onset and duration of tail-pinch eating, there is good evidence implicating dopamine as a key element in this behaviour.

In addition to dopamine, extensive pharmacological manipulation of serotonin metabolism has also been carried out (Antelman and Caggiula, 1977). In particular, the serotonin precursor 5-hydroxytryptophan attenuated tail-pinch eating. Tryptophan, when given alone, had no effect but antagonized the eating when injected in combination with the type A monoamine oxidase inhibitor clorgyline; in turn, pretreatment with PCPA reversed this effect. The further finding that the serotonin uptaker blocker Lilly 110140 reduced tail-pinch eating substantiates the argument for a modulatory influence of serotonin systems on stress-induced eating.

The finding that reductions in the synaptic activity of dopamine produce similar effects to the enhancement of activity at serotonergic synapses, suggests an interaction between dopamine and serotonin in the control of tail-pinch eating. Further experiments to establish a synergism between dopaminergic and serotonergic manipulations have supported the view that serotonin and dopamine interact reciprocally in the mediation of stress-induced eating (Antelman and Caggiula, 1977). Similar proposals for an interaction between these two amines in the control of feeding unrelated to stress have also been made (Blundell and Latham, 1978; Grossman, 1978) although it appears that tail-pinch eating is a most sensitive model for examining these relationships.

The power of the tail-pinch phenomena to discriminate between pharmacological treatments is illustrated by its influence on the action of anorexic drugs (Antelman et al., 1978). Amphetamine and methylphenidate failed to overcome eating induced by tail-pinch stress whereas fenfluramine produced an attenuation of this behaviour. The effective action of fenfluramine is in keeping with the effects of other serotonergic manipulations, while the failure of amphetamine is consistent with previous observations on dopamine metabolism. The sensitivity of tail-pinch-induced eating and its discriminatory power draw attention to its value in understanding the behavioural actions of drugs influencing feeding. In addition, this phenomena has further extended the theoretical base of feeding activities to embrace a hitherto unexplored aspect of eating. Tail-pinch eating is an intriguing example of stress-induced behaviour which has served as a test arena in the development of strategies for further pharmacological analysis of activation-induced feeding.

## D.  Self-selection of Nutrients

A large body of evidence indicates that animals possess the ability to select and to monitor qualitatively their intake of particular nutrients (Overmann, 1977). This phenomenon supports the idea that animals display specific hungers, and it follows that animals must have the capacity to associate the sensory qualities of foods with the consequences of their ingestion. This capacity has obvious adaptive value and represents a beneficial evolutionary strategy. A number of studies have shown that rats allowed to select from a cafeteria array of separate dietary components such as protein, fat, carbohydrate, vitamins and minerals are able to maintain a balanced intake of essential elements (e.g. Richter, 1943). In addition, this dietary self-selection can be influenced by the ambient temperature (Leshner et al., 1971), changing hormonal states (Leshner et al., 1972), activity level (Collier et al., 1969) and the availability of water (Overmann and Yang, 1973; Corey et al., 1978). Indeed, it appears that dietary self-selection is a fundamental characteristic of feeding behaviour in animals which becomes more clearly apparent when functional demands are placed on the system.

Until recently, this phenomenon had been ignored in pharmacological investigations of feeding in which animals are generally maintained on a single composite diet containing a balanced mixture of essential nutrients. However, interest in pharmacological aspects of voluntary self-selection has been promoted by theoretical developments concerning the role of neurotransmitter systems in the regulation of protein and carbohydrate intake. It has been proposed that the concentration of the transmitter serotonin in the brain is dependent upon the ratio of tryptophan to neutral amino acids in the plasma Fernstrom and Wurtman, 1974; Wurtman and Fernstrom, 1974). The nature of the diet exerts a major influence over this plasma ratio, and it has been demonstrated that a high carbohydrate meal can lead to increases in brain tryptophan and serotonin (Fernstrom and Wurtman, 1972). It has therefore been proposed that serotonin-containing brain neurons may function as "ratio-sensors": the rate of neurotransmitter synthesis in these neurons varying with the nutrient composition of the diet. Consequently, serotonin neurons could discriminate between the metabolic effects of various diets (Fernstrom and Wurtman, 1973). One implication of this process is that the feedback effect from neurotransmitter synthesis on feeding behaviour may involve qualitative rather than quantitative adjustments in food intake. This means that neurotransmitter activity will influence an animal's choice of nutrients. In keeping with this idea, Ashley and Anderson (1975) have demonstrated that in the weanling rat, the ratio of tryptophan to neutral amino acids in plasma is related to the amount of protein self-selected by the rat. In turn this has led to the suggestion that serotonin neurons participate in feeding not by regulating total calorie intake, but by controlling the balance of protein and carbohydrate in the diet.

This hypothesis lends itself readily to test by pharmacological agents and obliges experimenters to allow animals to self-select their intake of particular dietary components. This demand has led to the development of an experimental procedure in which animals are faced with two or more food containers holding varying concentrations of the major macro-nutrients protein, carbohydrate and fat. In a typical two-container design, animals are allowed to choose between 5 and 45%, or 15 and 55% isocaloric protein diets. Accordingly, by moderating their eating from a particular source, animals can adjust their elective consumption of protein and carbohydrate. In one of the first pharmacological studies using this paradigm, it was demonstrated that different anorexic drugs exerted distinctive effects on the pattern of selection (Wurtman and Wurtman, 1977). Fenfluramine and fluoxetine, which increase the synaptic activity of serotonin, displayed a protein sparing effect in weanling rats; that is, they reduced total food intake but actually increased the proportion of protein consumed. In contrast, amphetamine gave rise to an equal suppression of protein and total calorie intake. In an extension of this study using adult animals and allowing the rats to feed freely, fenfluramine maintained but did spare protein intake while amphetamine brought about a severe suppression of protein consumption (Blundell and McArthur, 1979).

More recently, it has been shown that the depletion of brain serotonin by systemic injections of para-chloro-phenyl alanine, intraventricular administration of 5, 7-dihydroxytryptamine or by electro-thermal lesions of the medial raphe nuclei lead to a selective decrease in protein intake (Ashley et al., 1979). In turn, this work is supported by the finding that drugs which are believed to enhance central serotonergic transmission selectively suppress carbohydrate consumption by rats (Wurtman and Wurtman, 1979). It is clear that the pharmacological manipulation of serotonin metabolism can bring about fairly orderly adjustments in the selection of macro-nutrients by rats although it remains to be demonstrated whether the primary effect is on protein or carbohydrate intake (Wurtman and Wurtman, 1979). This recent experimental work has illustrated the discriminatory power of the self-selection paradigm which should continue to be a crucial research device in the behavioural pharmacology of feeding.

## E. Micro-structural Analysis of Feeding Behaviour

In pharmacological experiments on feeding, one distinction which is often blurred is that between food intake and feeding behaviour. Food intake is a quantitative term which refers to the mass of nutrients consumed, whereas feeding behaviour draws attention to the qualitative aspects of an animal's movements as it satisfies its nutritional requirements. A measurement of food intake can be reduced to a single number, but feeding behaviour can only be described by reference to changes in state or to sequences of actions. For many animals, feeding is an episodic activity and even the eating episodes themselves show discontinuities in behaviour. In the rat or mouse, feeding behaviour can be characterized by continuously observing the behaviour of the animal and recording changes in activity. Using this procedure, Wiepkema (1971a) categorized and measured the particular episodes of eating (called bouts), the intervals of non-eating, and the relationship between these variables. In this way, qualitative changes in behaviour can be objectively represented. For example, following a period of food deprivation, Wiepkema found that the mean number of feeding bouts did not change; however the duration of these bouts was notably increased while the duration of the inter-bout intervals was decreased (Wiepkema, 1971b). This analytical technique can be used to characterize the effects of pharmacological manipulation on feeding. In turn, the drug-induced adjustments to the micro-structure of feeding behaviour can help to elucidate the way in which a drug enhances, or more commonly suppresses, food intake.

In a recent study employing this technique, the behaviour of rats during a 1 h-period was exhaustively recorded in six categories: eating, drinking, grooming, locomotor activity, resting and others. By means of a standard procedure for event recording, the observer noted the occurrence and the duration of all activities within the six categories provided by the schedule. From these records together with the food weighings, it is possible to derive the parameters of feeding shown in Table I.

*Table I*. Parameters of feeding derived from the analysis of the micro-structure of behaviour.

Total food intake (g)
Duration of time spent eating (min)
Latency (time elapsed before onset of eating) (min)
Number of eating bouts (n)
Size of bouts (g)
Duration of bouts (mins)
Local rate of eating (g/min)

It is worth noting that the measure of eating rate is a local value calculated only from the rat's actual eating time and is quite different from an overall rate which can be simply computed by dividing the weight of the food consumed by the duration of the testing period. The purpose of measuring these particular parameters is to permit the detection of certain subtle differences between the actions of drugs not revealed by a simple measure of the amount of food consumed. This can be demonstrated by considering the results of an experiment which compared the effects of equi-anorectic doses of amphetamine, fenfluramine, mazindol and diethylpropion. Although these compounds produced a similar suppression of food intake, they differed on a number of micro-structural parameters (Blundell and Latham, 1978). In particular, it was revealed that amphetamine markedly increased the latency to the initiation of eating, and actually caused rats to increase markedly the rate of consumption, an effect also displayed by mazindol. This finding was contrary to expectations, and is a phenomenon not normally associated with drugs which suppress food intake.

On the other hand, fenfluramine brought about a noticeable slowing of the rate of eating. It has since been demonstrated that this slow rate of eating is reliably displayed by drugs such as pimozide which block dopamine receptors and by compounds such as 5-hydroxytryptophan which enhance activity in serotonin systems (Blundell and Latham, 1978, 1979). However, it is clear that the slow rate of eating does not cause the reduction in food intake. For example, pimozide does not necessarily produce anorexia: when the rate of eating is slowed, the animals compensate by increasing the time spent eating resulting in no deficit in food intake. However, with a serotonergic drug such as fenfluramine, the rats do not compensate for the slow eating rate by increasing eating time. Consumption is curtailed independently of changes in the rate of eating (Blundell and Latham, 1980).

The power of the micro-analytical technique rests on the capacity to describe detailed behaviours displayed by animals when given the opportunity to feed. Eating can be blocked by a number of treatments which are quite unrelated to the processes through which an animal regulates its nutritional requirements. By closely observing the animal's actions, it is possible to decide whether eating is being constrained by a rational physiological process, or whether food intake is blocked by a contamination of the behaviour sequence. For example, a moderate dose of amphetamine alters many elements of the animal's feeding repertoire and disrupts the natural sequence of actions (Blundell and Latham, 1980). In this way, the technique can allow researchers to decide whether particular drugs can be useful tools to elucidate control mechanisms of feeding.

## VI. DRUG EFFECTS ON FREE-FEEDING BEHAVIOUR

### A. Continuous Monitoring of Feeding Patterns

The measurement of feeding patterns in free-feeding animals has gained wide acceptance as a useful tool for understanding the effects of various physiological and environmental manipulations on food intake. The power of the technique has been engendered by the apparent degree of stability observed in the free-feeding patterns of individual rats. In turn, this stability has prompted many investigators to apply sophisticated mathematical techniques in order to uncover the relationships that may exist between the various feeding parameters measured. Much of the work has centred around the measurement and extent of the relationships between meal size and pre- and post-meal intervals (Le Magnen, 1971; de Castro, 1975; Panksepp, 1973). To some degree, both the timing and the size of the meals taken by an individual rat reflect a complex interaction between its underlying physiological state and its behaviour in the testing environment.

The continuous monitoring of any behavioural activity poses problems of measurement and data reduction. Of the two, measurement poses the more fundamental problem since this provides the data for subsequent analysis. Food has been presented in a variety of forms; e.g. fluid, powder, blocks, precision pellets and diets with particular tastes, smells and textures. Furthermore, rats have been required to perform a variety of different behaviours including licking a drinkometer, traversing a tunnel for access to a food cup, performance of an operant such as a level press and removal of a pellet from a pellet-detecting eatometer. Both the physical properties of food and the behaviour required to acquire it have been shown to influence feeding patterns

(Balagura and Coscina, 1968; Collier, Hirsh and Hamlin, 1972; Levitsky, 1974). In addition, the testing environment itself has important effects on the patterning of feeding behaviour. In particular, lighting conditions are known to cause changes in the distribution and timing of meals (Borbely and Houston, 1974), and this has led some workers to argue that continuous low levels of illumination may reflect a more ecologically valid condition than the usual 12 h light–dark cycle (Panksepp and Ritter, 1975). Other factors known to influence feeding patterns are fluctuations in ambient temperature, experimenter intrusion and extraneous environmental noise.

Although certain methodological and theoretical issues remain unresolved, the application of continuous monitoring techniques to the investigation of pharmacological manipulations on food intake has revealed interesting and unexpected effects inaccessible to studies involving deprived rats (Blundell and Latham, 1978; Latham and Blundell, 1979). The following sections give a description of the continuous monitoring technique and subsequent data reduction as used in our laboratories.

## B. Testing Environment, Food Measurement and Data Acquisition

The testing environment used in our laboratories has been developed in order to eliminate the effects of extraneous variables. Accordingly, the animals' home cages are housed in sound attenuated, temperature controlled, ventilated experimental chambers. In turn, the experimental chambers are housed in a quiet, environmentally controlled laboratory. In order to minimize the effects of experimenter intrusion, routine maintenance of equipment, cleaning and experimental manipulation takes place every day during a 15-min period prior to lights off. Light in each chamber is provided by a 6 watt fluorescent tube mounted near the ventilator exhaust fan. The lights are programmed by an electrical timer to give a 12-h light–dark cycle.

Food in the form of 45 mg precision pellets is made available from a pellet-detecting eatometer located in each experimental chamber. The basic design is a modification of that used by Kissileff (1970) and consists of a Camden Instruments pellet dispenser connected to a V-shaped trough. The trough which is attached to the inside of the home cage (Fig. 4) has a light source and a photosensor positioned at opposite ends of the base of the V. Removal of the pellet by a rat activates the photosenor, completing the circuit which triggers the delivery of another pellet from the pellet dispenser. The arrival of the pellet again breaks the circuit. The whole cycle from pellet removal to replacement takes approximately 0.5 seconds and is well inside the ability of any rat to respond.

Coincident with the removal of a food pellet and activation of the pellet dispenser, a discrete pulse is sent to a NOVA 840 minicomputer situated in an adjacent room. At the interface of the computer, a unique line number corresponding to the experimental chamber from which the pulse was received, together with the current time of day to the nearest tenth of a second

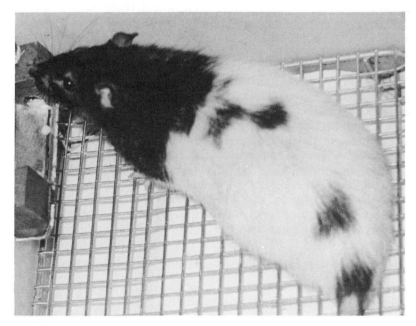

*Fig. 4.* Automated feeding trough used for the continuous monitoring of feeding.

is assigned. This information then passes to the computer buffer and is held until serviced by the data acquisition program which writes it to a floppy disk.

## C. Data Reduction

At the end of every 24-h monitoring period, the floppy disk can be changed and subsequently analysed on a NOVA 3 minicomputer. This allows acquisition of data to continue uninterrupted and also permits daily appraisal of experimental results. Several data analysis programs written in Data General Fortran IV have been developed in our laboratories. The main analysis program produces a printout in the form shown in Fig. 5. The new data can be stored indefinitely and, should changing theoretical consideration demand it, the data can be reanalysed. The data analysis presently performed in our laboratories can be divided into that related to meal size and the intervals between meals and that related to events within meals.

## D. Meals and Inter-meal Intervals

Possibly the major criterion in feeding pattern analysis is the definition of what constitutes a meal and parenthetically, what constitutes an inter-meal interval, since one determines the other. Since Richter's (1927) initial observations that rats appeared to feed in several distinct periods during a day's feeding, controversy has surrounded the adequacy of the criteria used to define episodes of feeding as meals. Most definitions of meals and inter-meal intervals have been gained from an intuitive appeal to the data, and in this respect our analysis is no different from many reported in the literature (Levitsky, 1970; de Castro, 1978). Attempts have been made to provide mathematically rather than intuitively derived criteria (Booth, 1972); however these have not led to any gain in conceptual clarity (Panksepp, 1978).

In the analysis of our own data, we have defined a meal as the removal of 5 or more 45 mg food pellets separated from any other number of 5 or more pellets by an interval of at least 15 min. The adequacy of the criteria we have chosen can only be substantiated by an appeal to the data analysis printout incorporating the criteria. The argument is obviously circular, however examination of feeding patterns derived from data using the above criteria leads us to believe that they are adequate. Figure 5 is an actual computer printout of the feeding pattern of a rat over a 2-day period. In this example, the first day (bouts 1–12) is the control day and the second (bouts 13–23) the experimental day. (In this case, the rat was injected intraperitoneally with a 5.0 mgKg$^{-1}$ solution of fenfluramine hydrochloride at the beginning of the second day.) Reading from left to right, we begin with the bout number (i.e. meal number). This identifies all the data associated with the meal and is useful for subsequent analysis. The second column indicates whether the meal was taken at night (N) or day (D). The next two columns give the actual start and end times of meals in decimal hours. A 24-h clock is used and zero corresponds to the start of the 12-h dark period. The fifth and sixth columns give the pre- and post-meal interval in decimal hours. Inspection of the post-meal intervals in this example shows them to vary between 0.32 to 3.92 h for bouts 1–12 on the control day. The great majority of these intervals are in excess of 1 h, however, the interval 0.32 h (20 min) following meal number 7 could be construed as an intra-meal interval so that meals 7 and 8 are in fact one meal. In defence of the criteria we have chosen, it can be shown that inter-meal intervals this small occur infrequently. An argument against considering such an interval as an intra-meal interval will be given in the next section. Columns eight and nine give the number of pellets and the weight in grams consumed during a meal; the next two columns give pre- and post-meal ratios.

Data corresponding to the control and experimental day are summarized at the bottom of Fig. 5. The first summary gives a comparison of the various feeding parameters and the second the distribution of meal sizes. Errors, at the foot of Fig. 5 represent the total number of pellets taken outside the criteria used for meals. It can be seen that out of a total of 950 pellets, only two pellets were taken outside of meals (i.e. less than 0.002%).

## E. Intra-meal Characteristics: Rates of Eating

The remaining sixteen columns of the eating data file (Fig. 5) are devoted to an examination of intra-meal events, and are based on an analysis of the interpellet

SLOT:1   ANIMAL:4      EATING    DATA   FILE:FENFB 5

| BOUT NO | START TIME | END TIME | INTERVAL PRE | INTERVAL POST | DURN SECS | NO. | WT. GM | W/I-RATIO PRE | W/I-RATIO POST | AVE. G/M | MON G/M | MON IPI | SIQ FMG | QUARTER-BOUT 1 | 2 | 3 | 4 MDN'S | QUARTER-BOUT IBI'S 1 | 2 | 3 | 4 | NO. | & SECS | DURN. |
|---|---|---|---|---|---|---|---|---|---|---|---|---|---|---|---|---|---|---|---|---|---|---|---|---|
| 1 N | 87 | 95 | 6 | 5 | 71 | 10 | 40 | 10 | 4 | 33 | 47 | 51 | 7 | 0 | 49 | 53 | 56 57 | 0 | 0 | 1 | 5 | 0 | 0 | 20 |
| 2 N | 329 | 336 | 81 | 233 | 278 | 47 | 188 | 23 | 19 | 39 | 42 | 56 | 11 | 59 | 53 | 56 | 63 55 | 11 | 0 | 0 | 0 | 1 | 21 | 0 |
| 3 N | 443 | 455 | 223 | 107 | 312 | 51 | 204 | 8 | 16 | 39 | 42 | 56 | 10 | 59 | 52 | 56 | 59 60 | 23 | 0 | 0 | 0 | 0 | 10 | 0 |
| 4 N | 707 | 721 | 107 | 252 | 399 | 66 | 264 | 24 | 16 | 39 | 42 | 57 | 8 | 59 | 57 | 70 | 64 | 184 | 3 | 2 | 6 | 2 | 32 | 9 |
| 5 N | 873 | 885 | 252 | 152 | 569 | 65 | 268 | 10 | 17 | 39 | 40 | 60 | 10 | 59 | 59 | 59 | 60 | 91 | 1 | 0 | 0 | 2 | 0 | 9 |
| 6 N | 1141 | 1149 | 152 | 258 | 421 | 67 | 268 | 17 | 19 | 38 | 40 | 60 | 8 | 58 | 58 | 61 | 60 | 12 | 0 | 1 | 0 | 0 | 32 | 20 |
| 7 N | 1141 | 1191 | 258 | 32 | 213 | 38 | 152 | 5 | 47 | 42 | 46 | 52 | 8 | 65 | 58 | 48 | 47 | 7 | 0 | 1 | 1 | 0 | 0 | 7 |
| 8 N | 1583 | 1593 | 32 | 392 | 316 | 46 | 184 | 5 | 7 | 34 | 36 | 65 | 8 | 66 | 61 | 61 | 65 | 9 | 1 | 0 | 1 | 6 | 0 | 9 |
| 9 N | 1848 | 1897 | 392 | 295 | 347 | 57 | 228 | 7 | 12 | 39 | 39 | 55 | 8 | 52 | 51 | 56 | 63 | 7 | 1 | 1 | 0 | 6 | 18 | 11 |
| 10 D | 2073 | 2065 | 295 | 176 | 329 | 57 | 229 | 12 | 11 | 41 | 42 | 57 | 14 | 55 | 54 | 65 | 57 | 18 | 1 | 1 | 2 | 14 | 22 | 7 |
| 11 D | 2073 | 2065 | 176 | 247 | 413 | 59 | 236 | 13 | 11 | 34 | 38 | 59 | 14 | 59 | 59 | 74 | 51 | 6 | 1 | 2 | 2 | 14 | 22 | 26 |
| 12 D | 2292 | 2310 | 247 | 194 | 606 | 72 | 288 | 13 | 14 | 28 | 34 | 62 | 17 | 68 | 68 | 65 | 69 | 23 | 2 | 2 | 14 | 17 | 3 | 75 |
| 13 N | 184 | 120 | 194 | 191 | 563 | 29 | 112 | 11 | 11 | 11 | 20 | 115 | 71 | 194 | 115 | 288 | 118 | 71 | 2 | 0 | 0 | 4 | 186 | 53 |
| 14 N | 221 | 226 | 103 | 103 | 327 | 12 | 48 | 4 | 4 | 8 | 12 | 191 | 167 | 0 | 0 | 0 | 0 | 156 | 1 | 1 | 29 | 1 | 48 | 35 |
| 15 N | 378 | 341 | 387 | 387 | 142 | 12 | 43 | 4 | 1 | 20 | 23 | 102 | 90 | 0 | 0 | 0 | 0 | 57 | 1 | 1 | 16 | 0 | 0 | 0 |
| 16 N | 728 | 727 | 223 | 223 | 336 | 24 | 68 | 1 | 3 | 12 | 34 | 70 | 9 | 0 | 0 | 0 | 0 | 45 | 1 | 1 | 12 | 0 | 0 | 184 |
| 17 N | 970 | 978 | 233 | 213 | 324 | 24 | 96 | 3 | 3 | 18 | 35 | 67 | 24 | 81 | 59 | 52 | 67 | 184 | 1 | 1 | 0 | 6 | 0 | 148 |
| 18 D | 1221 | 1222 | 243 | 52 | 431 | 52 | 208 | 8 | 40 | 28 | 32 | 73 | 13 | 84 | 69 | 85 | 70 | 101 | 1 | 1 | 8 | 1 | 30 | 0 |
| 19 D | 1284 | 1291 | 52 | 42 | 260 | 27 | 108 | 27 | 25 | 24 | 25 | 96 | 15 | 86 | 96 | 96 | 98 | 28 | 1 | 0 | 1 | 0 | 0 | 0 |
| 20 D | 1373 | 1339 | 527 | 527 | 206 | 29 | 116 | 2 | 2 | 31 | 32 | 74 | 10 | 70 | 70 | 74 | 53 | 10 | 1 | 1 | 8 | 0 | 0 | 0 |
| 21 D | 1866 | 1876 | 245 | 527 | 326 | 41 | 164 | 3 | 6 | 30 | 32 | 75 | 7 | 77 | 77 | 65 | 81 | 12 | 1 | 1 | 9 | 0 | 0 | 11 |
| 22 D | 2121 | 2127 | 245 | 245 | 222 | 36 | 144 | 5 | 13 | 38 | 38 | 62 | 8 | 52 | 52 | 67 | 73 | 14 | 1 | 0 | 14 | 0 | 0 | 7 |
| 23 D | 2215 | 2244 | 169 | 77 | 296 | 37 | 148 | 13 | 19 | 34 | 34 | 69 | 6 | 69 | 69 | 69 | 58 | 47. | 0 | 1 | 0 | 0 | 0 | 76 |

| DAY NO | NIGHT-TIME BOUTS NO | AV.WT. | AV.RTE | DAY-TIME BOUTS NO | WT. | AV.WT. | AV.RTE | OVER WHOLE DAY NO. | WT. | SIG | AV.WT | AV.RTE | NT:DY RATIOS NO. | WT. | TTL FDGS | UNIT SIZE | WT/GAP-RATIO PRE- | POST |
|---|---|---|---|---|---|---|---|---|---|---|---|---|---|---|---|---|---|---|
| 1 | 8 | 1560 195 | 41 | 4 | 500 | 245 | 39 | 12 | 2540 | 211 | 41 | 20 | 15 | 635 | 40 | 15 | 13 |
| 2 | 5 | 372 74 | 24 | 6 | 888 | 148 | 32 | 11 | 1268 | 114 | 28 | 8 | 4 | 315 | 40 | 8 | 11 |

MEAL-SIZE DISTRIBUTION - TOTALS & % BY WT.

|  | 0-19 | 20-39 | 40-59 | 60-79 | 80-99 | 100-119 | 120-139 | 140+ |
|---|---|---|---|---|---|---|---|---|
|  | 1 / 2 | 1 / 6 | 6 / 59 | 4 / 43 | 0 / 0 | 0 / 0 | 0 / 0 | 0 / 0 |
|  | 3 / 13 | 6 / 57 | 2 / 30 | 0 / 0 | 0 / 0 | 0 / 0 | 0 / 0 | 0 / 0 |

ERRORS= 2

*Fig. 5.* Example of a computer printout of data from two days of continuous monitoring of feeding. This eating data file displays the exact start and finish of every meal, the duration and size of each meal, various rates of eating during the meals, pre- and post-meal ratios and summaries of each day's data. In this example, the animal received a control injection on the first day and fenfluramine (5.0 mg kg⁻¹) on the second. The drug clearly reduced meal size and the rate of eating (see text for full explanation).

intervals. Before the introduction of computer-based analysis techniques in our laboratory, it was usual to give only a crude rate of eating. This was based on the amount of food consumed during a meal divided by the duration of the meal. This is still computed and is given as the average grams per minutes (AVE. G/M) in hundredths of a gram. However, not all interpellet intervals represent the amount of time between acquisition of the pellet, its consumption and acquisition of the next pellet.

Occasional large intervals may occur which represent intra-bout rather than interpellet intervals. These may be due to the rat adjusting its feeding position, grooming, scratching, drinking or its reactions to some external stimuli. The influence of these large infrequent intervals can be eliminated by the adoption of a median rate of eating. This is computed from the weight of food consumed in a meal, divided by the median interpellet interval (MDN. G/M in hundredths of a gram in Fig. 5). The median interpellet interval which is given to the nearest tenth of a second in Fig. 5 is computed from all of the interpellet intervals occurring within a meal. In addition, a measure of its variability in the form of the semi-interquartile range is also computed (SIQ. RN8 in tenths of a second). Quarter-bout medians are also computed as there is evidence in the literature that feeding rates may be higher at the start of meals and lower at the end (Wiepkema, 1971; Le Magnen, 1971). Indeed, the rate of eating, calculated from the median interpellet interval is slower over the second half of the meal than the first (Blundell and Latham, unpublished data).

Certain pharmacological manipulations have also been shown by us to decrease feeding rate. Drugs increasing serotonin metabolism lead to a decrease in meal size and a decrease in the rate of eating (Blundell and Latham, 1978) with the notable exception of the serotonin precursor tryptophan which, although it reduces meal size, has no effect on feeding rate (Latham and Blundell, 1979). Drugs blocking dopamine receptors (e.g. pimozide, $\alpha$-flupenthixol) actually lead to an increase in meal size and a reduction in feeding rate (Blundell and Latham, 1978). These data amply demonstrate that the rate of eating is not simply determined by hunger or developing satiety.

To further characterize feeding rate, we have used the technique of plotting log survivor functions of interpellet intervals. A log survivor function is displayed by plotting the intervals between behavioural events, in this case interpellet intervals, semilogarithmically. On the graph of a log survivor function, the abscissa corresponds to time "t" and the ordinate displays the log of the number of intervals whose lengths are greater than time "t" (see Cox and Lewis, 1966). In the example given (Fig. 6), we have given the log of percentage survivors so that a direct comparison can be made between the control and experimental conditions. Changes in the slope of a log survivor function indicate a change in the probability of an event occurring. Thus under the control condition (Fig. 6 upper section) there is a low probability of interpellet intervals greater than 15 sec occurring, over 95% of interpellet intervals falling between 3 and 8 sec (dark period). Under the experimental, fenfluramine conditions, there is a high probability of interpellet intervals greater than

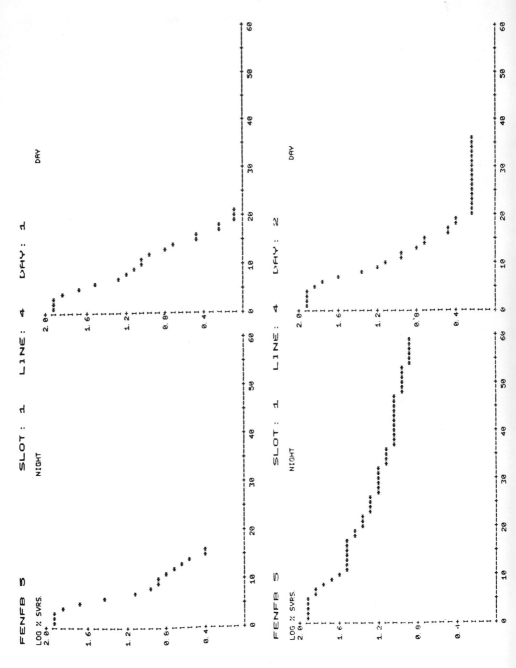

*Fig.* 6. Example of computer printouts of log survivor plots of interpellet intervals after saline treatment (top section) and fenfluramine (bottom). The drug has notably increased the size of the interpellet intervals (reduced the rate of eating) during the night-time period. The injections were made at the beginning of the dark phase.

15 sec occurring, only approximately 70% of interpellet intervals fall between 5 and 10 sec (dark period). Comparison of the slopes for the light period indicates a return to normal.

In order to determine where intra-meal intervals occur during meals reference can be made to the complete interpellet interval printout, however for ease of identification, it is also possible to display this on the eating file printout (Fig. 5). The last eight columns give information on the number of intra-bout intervals in each quarter of the meal together with the total time in seconds. The times are computed for any interpellet interval that exceeds twice the median interpellet interval. From this time, the median interpellet interval is subtracted, since this represents the time for eating, and the remainder is displayed in the table. Inclusion of this table in the mean eating file printout enables quick identification of the distribution of intra-meal intervals during the meal and together with the post-meal interval data provides information for validation of the 15 min inter-meal criterion.

## F. Time Course of Drug Effects

The continuous monitoring of feeding provides a detailed record of moment-to-moment adjustments in eating brought about by pharmacological treatment. However, the power of this analysis may be weakened by collapsing data over long time periods. Over the course of a 12- or 24-h period, a drug may rise to a peak concentration in blood (and other tissues), and the levels will then decline reflecting the half-life of the compound. In eating following a period of deprivation, it has been useful to compare the time course of changes in food intake with the time course for drug concentration in blood (Blundell et al., 1975). This can be achieved with great ease when feeding is continuously monitored. Figure 7 shows the temporal fluctuations over a 24-h period plotted in 2-h blocks. The parameters shown are average food intake, meal size, meal frequency and the intra-meal rate of eating following an injection of fenfluramine (5.0 mg kg$^{-1}$) at zero hours. It can be seen that food intake is suppressed for the first 12 h (dark period) after which there is little difference between the control and drug profiles. However, the drug profile does not display compensation in the second half of the day. The course of action of the drug on meal size and intra-meal rate of eating can also be traced, and although these profiles display certain similarities, it is clear that these two parameters can be disengaged.

At the present time, continuous monitoring of free-feeding patterns has only been sparingly used for the 24 pharmacological analysis of feeding (Blundell et al., 1976; Blundell and Latham, 1978, 1979; Burton et al., 1981; Latham and Blundell, 1979; Drewnowski and Grinker, 1978; Grinker et al., 1980). However, the sensitivity of the technique to drug manipulations together with the capacity to provide temporal profiles of changes in feeding parameters suggests that the procedure will become established as a powerful tool in the behavioural pharmacology of feeding.

## (7a) FOOD INTAKE

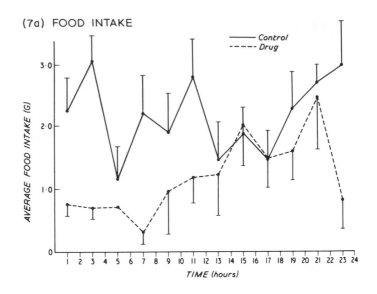

## MEAL FREQUENCY

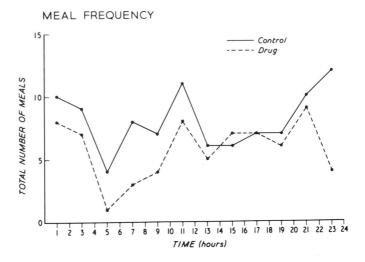

*Fig.* 7. Temporal profiles of feeding parameters following treatment with saline or fenfluramine (5.0 mg kg$^{-1}$). The data are plotted in 2-h blocks over a 24-h period. The time courses allow inspection of the degree of association and disengagement between different parameters (see text for comment).

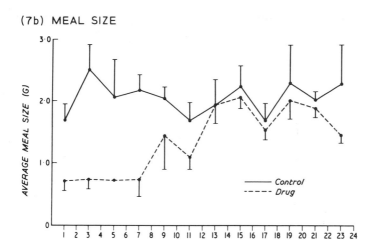

(7b) MEAL SIZE

AVERAGE MEAL SIZE (G)

——— Control
- - - - Drug

TIME (hours)

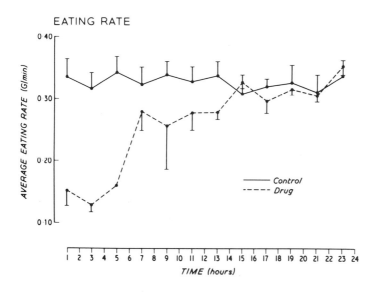

EATING RATE

AVERAGE EATING RATE (G/min)

——— Control
- - - - Drug

TIME (hours)

# VII. BEHAVIOURAL PHARMACOLOGY AND THE BIO-GRAMMAR OF FEEDING

Food intake is considered by many researchers to be a simple manifestation of an organism's need capable of easy measurement and quantification. In fact, feeding is a complex expression of a relationship between an animal's biological (under the skin) and social (beyond the skin) environment. Feeding behaviour is one of those activities which act as adhesives in forming an intimate bond between organisms and the world in which they live. In this sense, feeding is a special form of *transaction*, for organisms not only interact with the external environment containing food materials; they actually consume the environment which then forms part of the internal system. This is a delicate and complicated process. The puzzle is that on the one hand, feeding appears to be an automatic extension of a bodily need into the external world, and on the other hand, a diverse set of actions which fluctuate from moment to moment and from place to place.

One way to resolve this puzzle is to consider a grammar of feeding based on the idea of deep and surface structures such as that proposed for understanding language (Chomsky, 1965). The surface structure of feeding would vary according to the imposed environmental circumstances, but the deep structure or syntax would remain relatively constant. It follows that the surface structure, which may be considered as a dialect of eating, although dependent upon the deep structure, is subject to a wide variety of influences. Using this model, two weaknesses have become apparent in the behavioural pharmacology of feeding. First, changes in the surface structure induced by drugs have invariably been interpreted as actions upon the deep structure. Secondly, only limited attention has been given to the complexity of the surface structure. Just as very little would be known about language by counting the number of utterances produced, so only restricted information can be gathered about feeding by counting the number of grams ingested.

In addition to these provisions, certain studies of drugs on food intake have led to premature explanations in terms of the processes of hunger, appetite and satiety. Generally, these terms are used fairly loosely and it is often a matter of personal preference whether a decrease in food intake is interpreted as arising from a suppression of hunger or an enhancement of satiety. Similarly, it is a moot point whether increases in food intake represent increased hunger or defective satiety. It would be helpful to researchers if these terms were used with greater precision (to refer to consistent and distinctive adjustments in behaviour) or if the terms were abandoned in favour of a purely behavioural description of events. Figure 8 illustrates one way of conceptualizing the surface structure of eating in conjunction with the constructs frequently chosen to describe these events. In this conceptualization, hunger primarily determines the onset of eating and exerts a smaller effect on the amount eaten. Appetite is intimately linked to the sensory qualities of food and has a primary effect on the commodities selected and the amount consumed. Satiation refers to the process of bringing a meal to a close while satiety connotes the state of

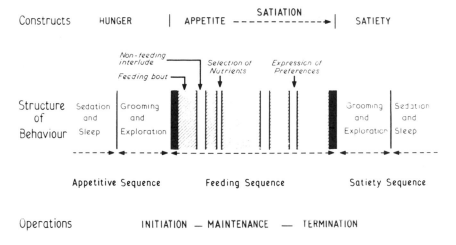

*Fig. 8.* Conceptualization of the structure of feeding behaviour showing the relationship between the expression of particular activities and constructs used to describe changes in intake. This plan may be useful in considering the mechanisms through which drugs enhance or suppress ingestion.

inhibition over further eating.

Using this conceptualization, it may be questioned how drug-induced changes in food intake should be interpreted. Since most of the catalogued effects of drugs on feeding indicate a suppression, rather than an enhancement of intake, it is worthwhile considering the possible explanations for an observed inhibition of food ingested. Table II indicates some of the effects related to the natural system regulating an animal's nutritional requirements and some non-specific effects. Inspection of these possible explanations suggests that it is far from easy to identify the cause of drug-induced suppression of eating from mere observation of the amount consumed. However, additional information derived from measured changes in the structure of behaviour, temporal patterns of feeding, selection of nutrients or manifest preferences for particular commodities will increase a researcher's confidence in the deduced explanation.

## A.  Amphetamine Anorexia: A Test Case

For more than forty years, it has been tacitly assumed by many researchers that the suppressive effect of amphetamine on food intake represents an interaction of this drug with mechanisms controlling food intake in response to nutritional requirements. The evidence for this belief is very weak and the appropriate conclusion after many years of research must be that the mechanism of amphetamine anorexia is still uncertain. Despite this lack of understanding, amphetamine has come to be regarded as a reference drug in the pharmacological study of anorexia. Moreover, pharmacological treatments which attenuate

*Table II*. Observed decrease in amount of food ingested. Possible explanations which could be invoked to account for drug-induced inhibition of food intake.

| Inhibition of food intake | |
|---|---|
| Feeding-related explanations | Non-specific explanations |
| (1) Decrease in requirement for calories | (1) Displacement of eating by increase in other normal activities |
| (2) Attempt to reduce intake of particular nutrients | (2) Inability to articulate motor movements of eating |
| (3) Shift in preferences for taste, texture, etc. | (3) Interference with ordering of feeding and non-feeding bouts within a meal |
| (4) Alteration in circadian pattern of ingestion | (4) Introduction of abnormal behaviours into the feeding repertoire |
| (5) Adjustments to the initiation, maintenance or termination of eating episodes | (5) Disruption of the appetitive sequence leading up to a meal |
| (6) Effect on hunger, appetite, satiation or satiety | (6) Creation of an internal physiological state inappropriate to ingestion |
| (7) Action on neural mechanism responsible for expression of calorie requirement | (7) Deflection of attention to non-salient features of the environment |

amphetamine anorexia are often used as evidence for the role of a particular transmitter in the control of normal feeding. It is worth pointing out that until the mechanism underlying the suppression of intake by amphetamine is elucidated, the drug will have limited use as a tool to explore natural controls of ingestion. However, the drug can of course be used as a tool to investigate the experimental suppression of feeding.

Amphetamine is an intriguing drug which produces a wide variety of effects on feeding. Eating is easily suppressed at high doses, but this is likely to be due, at least in part, to the introduction of stereotyped patterns of activity incompatible with the expression of eating. This action will be exacerbated by the use of severe periods of deprivation which are known to intensify stereotypy. Moderate doses of amphetamine lead to alterations in the ordering of general behaviour sequences (Norton, 1975) and to adjustments in the sequence of feeding activities (Burridge, 1980). These doses generally increase the rate of eating while reducing overall intake. Low doses of the drug may produce a decrement in feeding not related to the contamination of behaviour (Blundell and Burridge, 1979). However, doses of this magnitude are not widely used in studies on experimental anorexia. Consequently, much of the data on amphetamine and food intake may be only weakly related to the question of natural feeding processes. In addition, amphetamine has been shown to produce paradoxical increases in food consumption. This has been observed with doses of the drug in free-feeding animals (Blundell and Latham, 1978; Doggett and Dobrzansky, 1978), in animals subjected to lateral hypothalamic lesions (Stricker and Zigmond, 1976; Wolgin *et al.*, 1976), and occasionally in food-deprived animals (Holtzman, 1974). Amphetamine also has a severe suppressive effect on protein intake and fails to attenuate stress-induced eating. This constellation of effects suggests that a complex network of mechanisms is required to describe the effect of amphetamine on food intake. The actions will vary with the dose of the drug and with other features of the experimental circumstances. It seems appropriate that the effects of amphetamine on feeding should be interpreted cautiously, and that it would be wise to displace amphetamine as the reference compound in the pharmacology of anorexia. When the mechanisms underlying "amphetamine anorexia" are finally understood, there will have been a major advance in the behavioural pharmacology of feeding.

## B. The Next Ten Years

The last decade has seen important developments in the sensitivity and precision of pharmacological techniques. Specific agonists and antagonists have become available together with histochemical and biochemical tools to probe the action of drugs on neural tissue. In comparison, there has been a relative lag in the development of more intricate behavioural procedures. Accordingly, in considering the relationship between behaviour and pharmacology an imbalance in technology and sophistication is apparent. What is required in the behavioural pharmacology of feeding is a greater emphasis on *behaviour*. This should involve not only giving greater attention to the qualitative features of feeding and the environmental circumstances under which animals are expected to eat, but also to the bio-psychological conceptualization of feeding as a transaction between the biological and social domains. Pharmacological tools, used cautiously, can help to elucidate the bio-grammar of feeding.

## REFERENCES

Antelman, S. and Caggiula, A. R. (1977). Tales of stress-related behaviour: a neuro-pharmacological model. *In* "Animal models in psychiatry and neurology" (I. Hanin and E. Usdin, eds), Pergamon Press, New York.

Antelman, S. M. and Szechtman, H. (1975). Tail pinch induces eating in sated rats which appears to depend on striatal dopamine. *Science* **189**, 731–733.

Antelman, S. M, Szechtman, H., Chin, P. and Fisher, A. E. (1975). Tail-pinch induced eating, gnawing and licking behaviour in rats: dependence on the nigro-striatal dopamine system. *Brain Research* **99**, 319.

Antelman, S. M., Caggiula, A. R., Black, C. A. and Edwards, D. J. (1978). Stress reverses the anorexia induced by amphetamine and methylphenidate but not fenfluramine. *Brain Research* **143**, 580–585.

Ashley, D. V. M. and Anderson, G. H. (1975). Correlation between the plasma tryptophan to neutral amino acid ratio and protein intake in the self-selecting weanling rat. *J. Nutrition* **105**, 1412–1421.

Ashley, D. V. M., Coscina, D. V. and Anderson, G. H. (1979). Selective decrease in protein intake following brain serotonin depletion. *Life Sci.* **24**, 973–984.

Balagura, S. and Coscina, D. V. (1968). Periodicity of food intake in the rat as measured by an operant response. *Physiol. Behav.* **3**, 641–643.

Belluzi, J. D. and Stein, L. (1977). Enkephalin may mediate euphoria and drive reduction reward. *Nature* **266**, 556–558.

Bernier, A., Sicot, N. and Le Douarec, J. C. (1969). Action comparée de la Fenfluramine et de l'Amphétamine chez les rats obèse hypothalamiques. *Rev. Franc. d'Etudes Clin. et Biol.* **14**, 762–772.

Blundell, J. E. (1977). Is there a role for serotonin (5-hydroxytryptamine) in feeding? *Int. J. Ob.* **1**, 15–42.

Blundell, J. E. (1979). Serotonin and Feeding. *In* "Serotonin in Health and Disease" (W. B. Essman and L. Valzelli, eds.), pp. 403–449. Spectrum, New York.

Blundell, J. E. (1980). Hunger, appetite and satiety—constructs in search of identities. *In* "Lifestyles in Nutrition" (M. R. Turner, ed.), Applied Sci. Pub., London, pp. 21–42.

Blundell, J. E. and Burridge, S. L. (1979). Control of feeding and the psychopharmacology of anorexic drugs. *In* "The Treatment of Obesity", J. Munro, ed.), pp. 53–84. Lancaster MTP Press.

Blundell, J. E. and Latham, C. J. (1978). Pharmacological manipulation of feeding: possible influences of serotonin and dopamine on food intake. *In* "Central Mechanisms of Anorectic Drugs" (R. Samanin and S. Garattini, eds), pp. 83–109. Raven Press, New York.

Blundell, J. E. and Latham, C. J. (1979). Serotonergic influences on food intake: effect of 5-hydroxytryptophan on parameters of feeding behaviour in deprived and free-feeding rats. *Pharmacol. Biochem. Behav.* **11**, 431–437.

Blundell, J. E. and Latham, C. J. (1980). Characterization of the behavioural changes underlying the effects of amphetamine and fenfluramine on food consumption, and the antagonism by pimozide and methergoline. *Pharm. Biochem. Behav.*, **12**, 717–722.

Blundell, J. E., Latham, C. J. and Leshem, M. B. (1976). Differences between the anorexic action of amphetamine and fenfluramine: possible effects on hunger and satiety. *J. Pharm. Pharmacol.* **28**, 471–477.

Blundell, J. E. and McArthur, R. A. (1979). Investigation of food consumption using a dietary self-selection procedure: effects of pharmacological manipulation and feeding schedule. *Brit. J. Pharmac.*, **67**, 436–438P.

Blundell, J. E. and Rogers, P. J. (1978). Pharmacological approaches to the understanding of obesity. *Psychiat. Clin. N. Amer.* **1**, 629–650.

Blundell, J. E. and Rogers, P. J. (1980). Pharmacological manipulation as a tool to investigate human feeding processes: effects of anorexic drugs on food intake, food selection and preferences, hunger motivation and subjective experiences. *Appetite* **1**, (in press).

Blundell, J. E., Strupp, B. J. and Latham, C. J. (1977). Pharmacological manipulation of hoarding: Further analysis of amphetamine isoners and pimozide. *Physiol. Psychol.* **5**, 462–468.

Blundell, J. E., Campbell, B., Leshem, M. B. and Tozer, R. (1975). Comparison of the time course of the anorexic effects of amphetamine and fenfluramine with drug levels in blood. *J. Pharm. Pharmacol.* **27**, 187–192.

Booth, D. A. (1972). Some characteristics of feeding during streptozotocin-induced diabetes in the rat. *J. Comp. Physiol. Psychol.* **80**, 238–249.

Booth, D. A. (1976). Approaches to feeding control. *In* Appetite and Food Intake, (T. Silverstone, ed.) Abakon, Berlin.

Borbely, A. A. and Houston, J. P. (1974). Effects of two hour light–dark cycles on feeding, drinking and motor activity in the rat. *Physiol. Behav.* **13**, 795–802.

Bray, G. (1978). Intestinal bypass surgery for obese patients: behavioural and metabolic considerations. *Psychiat. Clin. N. Amer.* **1**, 673–690.

Burridge, S. B. (1980). Psychopharmacological investigation of some mechanisms underlying the inhibition of food intake in the rat with particular reference to amphetamine anorexia. Ph.D. Thesis, University of Leeds.

Burridge, S. B. and Blundell, J. E. (1979). Amphetamine anorexia: antagonism by typical but not atypical neuroleptics. *Neuropharmacol.* **18**, 453–457.

Burton, M. J., Cooper, S. J. and Potterwell, D. A. (1981). The effect of fenfluramine on the microstructure of feeding and drinking in the rat. *Br. J. Pharmac.* **72**, 621–633.

Chomsky, N. (1965). "Aspects of the Theory of Syntax". MIT Press, Cambridge, Mass.

Collier, G., Hirsch, E. and Hamlin, P. H. (1972). The ecological determinants of reinforcement in the rat. *Physiology and Behaviour* **9**, 705–716.

Collier, G., Hirsch, E. and Kanarek, R. (1977). The operant revisited. *In* Handbook of Operant Behaviour (W. K. Honig and J. E. R. Staddon, eds), Prentice Hall, New Jersey.

Collier, G., Leshner, A. and Squibb, R. (1969). Dietary self-selection in active and non-active rats. *Physiol. Behav.* **4**, 79–82.

Corey, D. T., Walton, A. and Wiener, N. I. (1978). Development of carbohydrate preference during water rationing: A specific hunger? *Physiol. Behav.* **20**, 547–552.

Cox, D. R. and Lewis, P. A. W. (1966). "The Statistical Analysis of Series of Events". Methuen, London.

Curzon, G., Joseph, M. H. and Knott, P. (1972). Effects of immobilization and food deprivation on rat brain tryptophan metabolism. *J. Neurochem.* **19**, 1967–1974.

De Castro, J. M. (1975). Meal pattern correlations: facts and artifacts. *Physiol. Behav.* **15**, 13–15.

De Castro, J.M. (1978). An analysis of the variance in meal patterning. *Neurosci. and Biobehav. Rev.* **2**, 301–309.

Dobrzanski, S. and Doggett, N. S. (1976). The effects of (+)-amphetamine and fenfluramine on feeding in starved and satiated mice. *Psychopharmacol.* **48**, 283–286.

Drewnowski, A. and Grinker, J. A. (1978). Food and water intake and meal and activity patterns of obese and lean Zuckers following chronic and acute treatment with $\Delta^9$ tetahydrocannabinol. *Pharmac. Biochem. Behav.* **9**, 619–630.

Epstein, A. N. (1959). Suppression of eating and drinking by amphetamine and other drugs in normal and hyperphagic rats. *J. Comp. Physiol. Psychol.* **52**, 37–45.

Fernstrom, J. D. and Wurtman, R. J. (1972). Brain serotonin content: physiological regulation by plasma neutral amino acids. *Science* **178**, 414–416.

Fernstrom, J. D. and Wurtman, R. J. (1973). Control of brain 5-HT content by dietary carbohydrates. *In* "Serotonin and Behaviour", J. Barchas and E. Usdin, eds), pp. 121–128. Academic Press, New York and London.

Fernstrom, J. D. and Wurtman, R. J. (1974). Nutrition and the brain. *Scientific American* **230**, 84–91.

Friedman, G., Weingarten, L. A. and Janowitz, H. D. (1962). A screening method for the assessment of appetite suppressants. *Am. J. Clin. Nutrit.* **10**, 225–230.

Garcia, J., Hawkins, W. G. and Rusiniak, K. W. (1974). Behavioural regulation of the milieu interne in man and rat. *Science* **185**, 824–831.

Garrow, J. S. (1978). "Energy Balance and Obesity in Man". North Holland, Amsterdam.

German, D. C. and Bowden, D. M. (1974). Catecholamine systems as the neural substrate for intra-cranial self-stimulation: a hypothesis. *Brain Research* **73**, 381–419.

Goldstein, A. (1976). Opioid peptides (endorphins) in pituitary and brain. *Science* **193**, 1081–1086.

Grinker, J. A. Drewnowski, A., Enns, M. and Kissileff, H. (1980). Effects of d-amphetamine and fenfluramine on feeding patterns and activity of obese and lean Zucker rats. *Pharmac. Biochem. Behav.* **12**, 265–275.

Hamilton, C. L. (1964). Rat's preference for high fat diets. *J. Comp. Physiol. Psychol.* **58**, 459–460.

Hirsch, E. and Collier, G. (1974). The ecological determinants of reinforcement in the guinea pig. *Physiol. Behav.* **12**, 239–249.

Holtzman, S. (1974). Behavioural effects of separate and combined administration of naloxone and d-amphetamine. *J. Pharmacol. Exp. Therap.* **189**, 51–60.

Ingle, D. J. (1949). A simple means of producing obesity in the rat. *Proc. Soc. Exp. Biol. Med.* **72**, 604–605.

Jacobs, B. L. and Farel, F. B. (1971). Motivated behaviour produced by increased arousal in the presence of goal objects. *Physiol. Behav.* **6**, 473–476.

James, P., Davies, H. and Ravenscroft, C. (1980). Is food intake under physiological control in man? *In* "Nutrition and Lifestyles" (M. R. Turner, ed.), Applied Sci. Pub., St. Albans.

Kanarek, R. B. and Hirsch, E. (1977). Dietary-induced overeating in experimental animals. *Fed. Proc.* **36**, 154–158.

Keesey, R. E. (1978). Set points and body weight regulation. *In* "Obesity: Basic mechanisms and treatment". Psychiatric Clinics of N. America **1**, 523–543.

Kirby, M. J., Pleece, S. A. and Redfern, P. H. (1978). The effect of fenfluramine on obesity in rats—a new method for the screening of potential antiobesity agents. *Brit. J. Pharmacol.*

Kissileff, H. (1970). Free-feeding in normal and 'recovered lateral' rats monitored by a pellet detecting eatometer. *Physiol. Behav.* **5**, 163–173.

Lamb, M. E. (1975). Physiological mechanisms in the control of maternal behaviour in rats: a review. *Psychol. Bull.* **32**, 104–119.

Latham, C. J. and Blundell, J. E. (1979). Evidence for the effect of tryptophan on the pattern of food consumption in free-feeding and deprived rats. *Life Sci.* **24**, 1971–1978.

Le Magnen, J. (1971). Advances in studies on the physiological control and regulation of food intake. *In* "Progress in Physiological Psychology" (E. Stellar and J. M. Sprague eds), pp. 203–261. Academic Press, London and New York.

Le Magnen, J. and Tallon, S. (1966). La periodicitée spontanée de la prise d'aliments ad libitum du rat blanc. *J. Physiol.* (Paris), **58**, 323–349.

Leshner, A., Collier, G. and Squibb, R. (1971). Dietary self-selection at cold temperatures. *Physiol. Behav.* 1971**b**, 1–3.

Leshner, A., Siegel, A. and Collier, G. (1972). Dietary self-selection by pregnant and lactating rats. *Physiol. Behav.* **8**, 151–154.

Levitsky, D. A. (1974). Feeding conditions and intermeal relationships. *Physiol. Behav.* **12**, 779–787.

Margules, D. L., Moisset, B., Shibuya, H. and Pert, B. (1978). β-endorphin is associated with overeating in genetically obese mice (ob/ob) and rats (fa/fa). *Science* **202**, 988–991.

Miller, N. E. (1957). Experiments on motivation. *Science* **126**, 1271–1278.

Miller, N. E., Bailey, C. J. and Stevenson, J. A. F. (1950). Decreased 'hunger' but increased food intake resulting from hypothalamic lesions. *Science* **112**, 256–259.

Mills, M. J. and Stunkard, A. J. (1976). Behavioural changes following surgery for obesity. *Am. J. Psychiat.* **133**, 527.

Moran, G. (1975). Severe food deprivation: some thoughts regarding its exclusive use. *Psychol. Bull.* **82**, 543–557.

Mrosovsky, N. (1971). "Hibernation and Hypothalamus". Appleton-Century-Crofts, New York.

Mrosovsky, N. and Powley, T. L. (1977). Set points for body weight and fat. *Behav. Biol.* **20**, 205–223.

Norton, S. (1973). Amphetamine as a model for hyperactivity in the rat. *Physiol. Behav.* **11**, 181–186.

Overmann, S. and Yang, M. (1973). Adaptation to water restriction through dietary selection in weanling rats. *Physiol. Behav.* **11**, 781–786.

Panksepp, J. (1973). Reanalysis of feeding patterns in the rat. *J. Comp. Physiol. Psychol.* **82**, 78–94.

Panksepp, J. (1978). Analysis of feeding patterns: data reduction and theoretical implications. *In* "Hunger Models" (D. A. Booth, ed.), 144–166. Academic Press, London and New York.

Panksepp, J. and Ritter, M. (1975). Mathematical analysis of energy regulatory patterns of normal and diabetic rats. *J. Comp. Physiol. Psychol.* **89**, 1019–1028.

Perez-Cruet, J., Tagliamonte, A., Tagliamonte, P. and Gessa, G. L. (1972). Changes in brain serotonin metabolism associated with fasting and satiation in rats. *Life Sci.* **11**, 31–39.

Reynolds, R. W. (1959). The effect of amphetamine on food intake in normal and hypothalamic hyperphagic rats. *J. Comp. Physiol. Psychol.* **52**, 682–684.

Richter, C. P. (1927). Animal behaviour and internal drives. *Quart. Rev. Biol.* **2**, 307–343.

Richter, C. (1943). Total self-regulatory functions in animals and human beings. Harvey Lecture Series, **38**, 63–103.

Robbins, T. W. and Fray, P. J. (1980). Stress-induced feeding: fact or fiction? *Appetite*, (in press).

Rogers, P. J. and Blundell, J. E. (1980). Investigation of food selection and meal parameters during the development of dietary-induced obesity. *Appetite* **1**, 85.

Rossier, J., Rogers, J., Shibasaki, T., Guillermin, R. and Bloom, F. E. (1979). Opioid peptides and α-melanocyte-stimulating hormone in genetically obese (ob/ob) mice during development. *Proc. Nat. Acad. Sci.* **76**, 2077–2080.

Rozin, P. (1976). The selection of foods by rats, humans and other animals. *In* "Advances in the Study of Behaviour VI". (J. Rosenblatt, R. Hinde, C. Beer and E. Shaw, eds), pp. 21–76, Academic Press, New York and London.

Roszowski, A. P. and Kelley, N. M. (1963). A rapid method for assessing drug inhibition of feeding behaviour. *J. Pharm. Exp. Therap.* **140**, 367–374.

Rowland, N. E. and Antelman, S. M. (1976). Stress-induced hyperphagia and obesity in rats: A possible model for understanding human obesity. *Science*, **191**, 310–312.

Stark, P. and Totty, O. W. (1967). Effects of amphetamines on eating elicited by hypothalamic stimulation. *J. Pharm. Exp. Therap.* **158**, 272–278.

Schachter, S. (1971). Some extraordinary facts about obese humans and rats. *Amer. Psychol.* **26**, 129–144.

Schemmel, R., Mickelsen, O. and Tolgay, Z. (1969). Dietary obesity in rats: influence of diet, weight, age and sex on body composition. *Am. J. Physiol.* **216**, 373–379.

Sclafani, A. (1978). Dietary obesity. *In* "Recent Advances in Obesity Research" **II**, (G. Bray, ed.), pp. 123–132. Newman, London.

Sclafani, A., Koopmans, H. S., Vasselli, V. R. and Reichman, M. (1978). Effects of intestinal by-pass surgery on appetite, food intake and body weight in obese and lean rats. *Am. J. Physiol.* **234**, E389–E398.

Sclafani, A. and Kluge, L. (1974). Food motivation and body weight levels in hypothalamic hyperphagic rats: a dual lipostat model of hunger and appetite. *J. Comp. Physiol. Psychol.* **86**, 28–46.

Sclafani, A. and Springer, D. (1976). Dietary obesity in normal adult rats: similarities to hypothalamic and human obesity syndromes. *Physiol. Behav.* **17**, 461–471.

Stricker, E. M. and Zigmond, M. J. (1976). Recovery of function following damage to central catecholamine-containing neurons: a neurochemical model for the lateral hypothalamic syndrome. *In* "Progress in Physiological Psychology", (J. M. Sprague and A. N. Epstein, eds), Vol. 6, pp. 121–188. Academic Press, New York and London.

Sullivan, A. (1978). Novel pharmacological approaches to the treatment of obesity. *In* "Recent Advances in Obesity Research II", (G. Bray, ed.), pp. 442–452. Newman, London.

Sullivan, A. C., Triscari, J. and Spiegel, H. E. (1977). Metabolic regulation as a control for lipid disorders II. Influence of (−)-hydroxycitrate on genetically and experimentally induced hypertriglyceridemia in the rat. *Am. J. Clin. Nutrit.* **30**, 777–784.

Sullivan, A. C., Triscari, J., Hamilton, J. G. and Miller, O. N. (1974). Effect of (−)-hydroxycitrate upon the accumulation of lipid in the rat II. Appetite. *Lipids* **9**, 129–134.

Tedeschi, D. H. (1966). Pharmacological evaluation of anorectic drugs. *In* "Methods in Drug Evaluation", (P. Mantegazza and R. Piccinini, eds), pp. 341–350. North Holland, Amsterdam.

Thode, W. F. and Carlisle, H. J. (1968). Effect of lateral hypothalamic stimulation on amphetamine-induced anorexia. *J. Comp. Physiol. Psychol.* **66**, 547–549.

Thompson, T. and Schuster, C. R. (1968). "Behavioural Pharmacology". Prentice-Hall, Englewood Cliffs, N.J.

Valenstein, E. S., Cox, V. C. and Kakolewski, J. W. (1970). Re-examination of the role of the hypothalamus in motivation. *Psychol. Rev.* **77**, 16–31.

Waddington, C. H. (1977). "Tools for Thought". Paladin, St. Albans.

Wiepkema, P. R. (1971a). Behavioural factors in the regulation of food intake. *Proc. Nutrit. Soc.* **30**, 142–149.

Wiepkema, P. R. (1971b). Positive feedbacks at work during feeding. *Behaviour* **39**, 266–273.

Wise, R. A. (1978). Catecholamine theories of reward: a critical review. *Brain Research* **152**, 215–247.

Wise, R. A., Spindler, J., De Wit, H. and Gerber, G. J. (1978). Neuroleptic-induced 'anhedonia' in rats: pimozide blocks reward quality of food. *Science* **201**, 262–264.

Wirtshafter, D. and Davis, J. D. (1977). Set points, settling points and the control of body weight. *Physiol. Behav.* **19**, 75–78.

Wolff, F. W. (1976). Peripheral and Hormonal mechanisms—a group report. *In* "Appetite and Food Intake" (T. Silverstone, ed.). Abakon, Berlin.

Wolgin, D. L., Cytawa, J. and Teitelbaum, P. (1976). The role of activation in the regulation of food intake. *In* "Hunger: Basic Mechanisms and Clinical Implications". (D. Novin, W. Wyrwicka and G. Bray, eds, pp. 179–191. Raven Press, N. Y.

Wurtman, R. J. and Fernstrom, J. D. (1974). Effect of the diet on brain neurotransmitters. *Nut. Rev.* **32**, 193–200.

Wurtman, J. J. and Wurtman, R. J. (1977). Fenfluramine and fluoxetine spare protein consumption while suppressing caloric intake by rats. *Science* **198**, 1178–1180.

Wurtman, J. J. and Wurtman, R. J. (1979). Drugs that enhance central serotonergic transmission diminish elective carbohydrate consumption by rats. *Life Sci.* **24**, 895–904.

Yamamoto, W. S. and Brobeck, J. R. (1965). "Physiological Controls and Regulations". Saunders, Philadelphia.

# 4 □ Measurement of Hunger and Food Intake in Man

## T. Silverstone

### I. MEASUREMENT OF HUNGER

In contrast to the situation observed in other animals, it is only in man that we can actually ask how hungry a given individual is, and thus it is only in man that we can examine the effects of drugs on the subjective sensations underlying hunger. But although we can examine such effects, and may even begin to quantify them, we cannot really "measure them". When, for example, subjects are asked to score the severity of their hunger on a rating scale in which 0 = no hunger, 1 = mild hunger, 2 = moderate hunger and 3 = severe hunger, the actual score given by any one subject at any particular time is not necessarily equal to the same score given by another subject at a different time. Nor can we assume that a change in rating from say 3 to 1, is twice as great as that from 1 to 0. All that these instruments allow us to do is to observe the direction of change within an individual over a set time, and to compare it with respect to both direction and magnitude to the change occurring within that same individual over a set time. One way in which these two occasions may differ is whether or not a drug has been administered.

While such a relatively blunt scoring system as that just described can distinguish between the effects of drugs affecting appetite and inert placebo, provided these differences are large, for the recognition of more subtle effects on hunger, greater sensitivity in the method of rating is required. A method which meets these requirements for greater sensitivity is the visual analogue scale.

## A. Visual Analogue Scales

Visual analogue scales (VAS) are straight lines, usually 100 mm long, labelled with the extremes of the subjective feelings to be quantified (Aitken, 1969). For use in experiments involving hunger and food intake, a hunger VAS, one end of which is labelled "Not at all hungry", and the other end "As hungry as

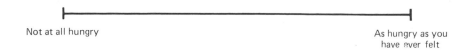

Not at all hungry                                          As hungry as you
                                                           have ever felt

*Fig. 1.* Visual analogue scale for hunger ratings.

you have ever felt" was found to be suitable (Silverstone and Stunkard, 1968), Fig. 1. Subjects are asked to mark the VAS at the point which they consider to be appropriate to their hunger sensations at the particular time they are completing it.

When subjects are presented with a succession of hunger VAS at fixed intervals, the pattern of their hunger response to a drug, or other experimental variable, can be evaluated. It is, as it were, a "hunger thermometer". However before any rating instrument, such as the hunger VAS, can be used in practice, it must be shown to be both reliable and valid.

### (1) *Reliability*
This refers to the property of reproducibility. For example: is change in the hunger ratings which occurs in response to a given drug in one group of subjects the same as occurs in a second group of subjects (assuming consistency of pharmacological activity)? That is, does the scale have reliability between different subjects? Secondly, does the same drug have the same effect on hunger ratings in the same subject on two different occasions? That is, does it have test–retest reliability? The hunger VAS has been shown to have both between-subject and test–retest reliability.

(a) *Between-Subject Reliability.* When testing the anorectic effect of a new potential anorectic agent, tiflorex, we found that the degree of subjective anorexia produced by the drug, as well as its time course of action, determined by changes in VAS ratings, was the same in two different groups of subjects (Silverstone and Fincham, 1978). More recently, we have found the same consistency in VAS response to a standard 10 mg dose of dexamphetamine sulphate (d-Amp) in different groups of subjects (Kyriakides and Silverstone, in preparation).

(b) *Test–Retest Reliability.* In a dose–response study of d-Amp, we have found that the same subjects showed similar dose-related responses to 10 and 20 mg d-Amp in hunger VAS ratings on two different occasions (Wells and Silverstone, in preparation). In a non-pharmacological experiment, Robinson *et al.* (1975) described within-subject consistency of VAS ratings during periods of food deprivation.

### (2) *Validity*
To ask whether or not any given measure is valid, is to ask whether it measures

what it is intended to measure. If, for example, we were examining the validity of a subjective scale of loudness, we could test its validity against objective physical measurements made with accurate sound metering instruments (Maxwell, 1978). However, such comparisons are not available to us in the field of hunger as there is no external objective standard against which we can compare it. All we are in a position to do is to see whether changes in hunger VAS ratings are accompanied by changes in food intake in the expected direction, and whether the magnitude of the VAS changes correspond to the magnitude of the changes in food intake. That is to say, if a subject rates himself as less hungry on one occasion than on another, does he eat correspondingly less on the first occasion than on the second?

Using a standard sandwich meal (see below) we found that a reduction of hunger VAS ratings produced by d-Amp in normal male subjects was closely paralleled by a reduction in food consumption (Silverstone and Stunkard, 1968). Similarly, we have shown that a d-Amp-induced reduction in hunger VAS scores determined 2 h after administration of the drug was followed by a significant reduction of food intake in the subsequent 2 h in normal female volunteers (Kyriakides and Silverstone, in preparation), Fig. 2. Similar comparisons between hunger VAS ratings and food intake were made by Robinson *et al.* (1975) in normal subjects and a population of psychiatric patients. Both groups showed a clear-cut relationship between hunger VAS and the amount of food consumed.

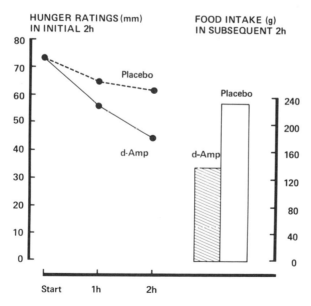

*Fig. 2.* The effect of a single oral dose of 10 mg dextroamphetamine on hunger ratings and on subsequent food intake in normal female subjects.

## B.  Questionnaires and Other Rating Scales

In a study to determine the effect of total starvation on subjective hunger, we developed a questionnaire designed to quantify the changes in hunger and in the desire to eat, which obese patients experienced during the course of 14 days total starvation (Silverstone *et al.*, 1966). This questionnaire included items on subjective hunger, the sensation of "emptiness" and how much they could eat. Gagnon and Tetreault (1975) adopted a similar approach in their study of the anorectic effects of d-Amp and fenfluramine (FF). Their questionnaire contained two five-point rating scales relating to how hungry the subjects had felt just before a meal eaten 4 h previously.

The relevant questions were:
(a) At the start of the meal, was your appetite very great, great, normal, small or absent?
(b) At the start of the meal, how hungry were you? Much more than usual, as usual, less than usual, much less than usual?

Even when used retrospectively, the questionnaire was able to detect significant differences between the active drugs and placebo, and to discern a dose–response effect; 60 mg FF lowered the hunger ratings more than either 20 or 40 mg. Furthermore, the reduction in hunger rating produced by both d-Amp and FF were associated with a corresponding reduction in food intake. More recently, Durrant and Royston (1979) have developed individualized hunger and appetite scales to take account of the considerable variation in the way hunger is experienced from one person to another (Monello *et al.*, 1965). They distinguished between hunger, which they defined as "physiological signals felt from inside the body", and appetite, which they defined as "mental signals indicating the desire to eat". Fixed five-point rating scales were used to quantify both hunger and appetite; the exact criteria for each point on any given patient's rating scale being decided upon after detailed consultation with that patient. The individualized hunger scale was shown to be highly sensitive to calorie dilution procedures; and although the appetite scale was not as sensitive as the hunger scale, there was a statistically significant correlation between the two. Furthermore, changes in hunger scores were significantly correlated to changes in salivation (see below).

## C.  Salivation

In his classical experiments on conditioned reflexes, Pavlov (1928) used the salivary response to the sight of food as a measure of an animal's desire to eat. He noted that such salivation could be affected by the nature of the food presented, and how long it had been since the dog had last eaten; the longer the period of deprivation, the greater the salivary response. On the basis of this and other reports, Wooley and Wooley (1973) suggested that the salivation response to the sight of food might be used as an objective measure of appetite in man. To do this, they placed standard, weighed dental wadding rolls into the subjects' mouths (one sublingually, two buccally bilaterally). The salivatory response was determined by weighing the rolls before and after being in the mouth for a standard time. The salivatory response to food-related stimuli in normal-weight subjects was found to increase with increasing degrees of food deprivation, and was subsequently found to be sensitive to manipulation of the calorie content of a "meal" given at a set time before the salivatory response was measured.

Unfortunately, this ingenious approach is probably not applicable to studies of drugs affecting appetite, as most of the relevant drugs have a direct autonomic action on the salivary glands themselves irrespective of any central effects such drugs might be having on hunger.

## D.  Conclusion

For short-term studies involving the determination of the effects of drugs on hunger, the most generally useful measure appears to be the hunger VAS. It is simple to complete, easy to score, and has been shown to be both reliable and valid. When used in conjunction with direct measures of food intake (see below) and plasma levels of the drug being investigated, a comprehensive profile of the anorectic (or orexigenic) potential of a given drug can be obtained.

## II.  MEASUREMENT OF FOOD INTAKE

As well as assessing the effect of a drug on subjective hunger ratings, it is equally important to be able to measure its effect on food consumption in man. For it is its effect on food consumption which largely, if not entirely, determines how the drug in question influences body weight, and it is the change in body weight produced by the drug which is generally its most significant effect in clinical terms. There are two approaches to measuring food intake in man; the indirect and the direct.

## (A)  Indirect Measures

### (1)  *Observations of Eating Behaviour*
Careful observation of an individual while he is eating can yield considerable information concerning his choice of food, his rate of eating, the time taken to finish a set portion of food, and the latency to start eating. Some of these parameters are more easily measured in certain situations than in others. For example, the recording of food choice is most appropriately done in a situation where the choice is wide, as for example in a cafeteria (Stunkard, 1977). However, to examine the more detailed features of eating, such as bite frequency, it is easier to observe subjects in a more scientific setting. Peering closely at an unsuspecting diner in a public restaurant, while surreptitiously jotting down repeated observations, is quite likely to be misinterpreted by the innocent subject, possibly leading to an unfortunate outcome! In any case it is

impossible, short of putting a drug in the drinking water, to undertake pharmacological investigations in public places. Such studies are best conducted in a laboratory setting with informed, consenting subjects. In recent years, the availability of video-tape recordings has greatly increased the reliability of such observations; the tapes can be viewed repeatedly and the measures checked for consistency. In the field of drug studies, Blundell *et al.* (1979) has successfully used this technique to compare the effects of FF to those of d-Amp on the latency to start feeding, on the rate of eating, on the choice of type of food selected (i.e. whether high protein or high carbohydrate) and on the time taken to complete a meal. It is, however, a time-consuming activity to scrutinize video-tapes sufficiently often to ensure accuracy, and two observers are usually required to ensure reliability.

### (2) *Diet Diaries*

A diet diary is a detailed record kept by the subject or patient of everything that he or she has consumed over a given period, and is usually completed once or twice each day. They are particularly useful in the longer-term assessment of the effects of drugs on food intake, especially if such observations are extended over days or weeks. When used with care, and regularly checked against independent observations of actual food intake, such measures can be reasonably reliable, and it has proved possible to use them to detect the effects of drugs on feeding (Silverstone *et al.*, 1968). However, there are considerable problems associated with this approach. First of all, it is very easy for a subject to forget exactly what he or she has eaten since last completing the diary; the record then becomes incomplete. Secondly, the sizes or portions given are usually only approximations, making exact calculations of total calorie intake impossible. However, by suitable training these sources of error can be lessened.

### (3) *Body Weight*

In the great majority of longer-term clinical studies involving drugs which influence appetite and food intake, it is body weight which is measured rather than appetite or food intake. The implicit assumption being made is that the changes in body weight which are observed are secondary to corresponding changes in hunger, and consequently to changes in food intake. While such an assumption is probably true in the majority of cases, it may not necessarily always be so. For example, a drug affecting appetite might also produce a loss of weight partly by increasing energy expenditure. In that case (and it has been suggested that at least one drug, FF, may act in this way) change in weight only partly reflects changes in hunger and food intake.

In those studies of anorectic drugs in which an attempt has been made to monitor food intake by means of diet diaries as well as measuring body weight, close correspondence was found between weight loss and reported reduction in food intake. A similar relationship between changes in reported food intake and body weight, although in the opposite direction, (an increase in body weight accompanied by an increase in food intake), has been observed with drugs which increase hunger such as cyproheptadine (Silverstone and Schuyler, 1975) and chlorpromazine (Robinson *et al.*, 1975). However in one of these studies, the relationship between changes in hunger ratings and changes in body weight, although in the appropriate direction, was not as close. This may well be because individuals vary much more in the way they estimate the experience of hunger than they do in the more familiar task of monitoring their food intake. Furthermore, a drug may have a greater effect on food intake than on hunger, as may be the case with FF in some circumstances (see Chapter 5).

## B. Direct Measures

### (1) *Liquid Nutrients*
In order to obtain a continuous and accurate measure of calorie intake in man, Hashim and Van Italie (1964) developed a technique whereby a human subject could obtain a measured quantity of a liquid nutrient of known calorie content delivered into his mouth by pressing a button. By incorporating a time-monitoring device into the machine, it proved possible to record a subject's nutrient intake on a minute-to-minute basis over an extended period. Normal subjects were found to be able to maintain a stable body weight over several days feeding only from the machine in spite of not being able to see how much they had consumed. Adapting this technique for shorter-term experiments, Jordan *et al.* (1966), used a hidden reservoir of liquid nutrient from which the subject sucked freely through a steel "straw" over a set time under constant conditions. The volume of nutrient ingested during fixed intervals was measured by an observer making readings from the calibrated reservoir (a 100 ml graduated burette). Subjects completed 9-point hunger rating scales before each test session, and at 5-min intervals during the ingestion period. A high correlation was found between subjective hunger ratings and the amount of nutrient ingested in the subsequent 5 min.

Pudel (1976), using a similar methodological approach, was able to show that ingestion of the liquid nutrient by normal subjects was sensitive to drug effects; fenfluramine led to a significant reduction in intake as compared to placebo. In spite of the great advantage of ease of measurement which these methods have, they also have significant limitations. In particular, the substitution of liquid nutrient for solid food means that it is drinking rather than eating that is measured (Warner and Balagura, 1975). Also, it is probably misleading to call such an instrument a "food dispensing apparatus" (Hashim and Van Italie, 1964) or to refer to its use as permitting "direct measurement of food intake" (Jordan *et al.*, 1966) or even to describe the behaviour observed as "experimental feeding" (Pudel, 1976). A further disadvantage which these methods have is in the monotony of nutrient provided; no element of choice is possible, and there is thus no opportunity for the subject to savour the variety of tastes and consistencies which occur during the course of a normal meal.

## (2) *Solid Food*

It is obviously less easy to quantify directly how much solid food is eaten over a given time in terms of calorie and weight than it is to measure the intake of a standardized liquid nutrient. This is particularly the case when there is a wide variety of choice of food. A number of methods have been devised to overcome this problem. As with many forms of clinical measurement, the proposed solutions are a compromise between accuracy of measurement on the one hand, and ease of application on the other.

(a) *Bomb Calorimetry of Duplicate Meals*. This is the most accurate of all the available methods for determining calorie consumption at a given meal. In this technique, two identical duplicate meals are prepared with weighed and measured constituents. The subject is asked to eat his fill from one of the two duplicate meals and what is left is placed in a bomb calorimeter; its calorie content is then measured. The calorie content of the untouched duplicate is similarly measured; the difference between the two is equivalent to the calories consumed by the subject. This method requires a painstaking eye to detail by an expert dietitian and is thus both time consuming and expensive. Furthermore, its use is limited to studies involving only one or two subjects at a time. In most circumstances, such constraints are likely to outweigh the advantage of verisimilitude which this method has.

(b) *Standardized Foods*. At the other extreme are those methods in which the intake of standardized foods is measured. For this purpose, nuts (Schachter, 1971) and crackers (Price and Grinker, 1973), or manufactured (and therefore presumably standardized) foods such as pieces of sausages (Warner and Balagura, 1975) have been used. While it is indeed a simple procedure to count how many crackers, nuts or pieces of sausage have been eaten, the foods themselves are more in the nature of snacks than complete meals, and they can hardly be administered as the sole source of energy over a period of longer than an hour or two. A further drawback which they share with liquid nutrients, is the lack of variety inherent in their use.

(c) *Sandwich Meals*. In an attempt to combine ease of measurement with a certain amount of variety in as naturalistic a setting as possible, we developed a standardized sandwich meal (Silverstone and Stunkard, 1968). At such a meal, subjects are given a plate containing a predetermined number of quartered sandwiches with the crusts removed. The subjects are instructed to eat as many of these almost bite-sized aliquots of food as they like in a given time. After they have finished eating, the number of each variety of quartered sandwich is calculated from the number remaining; and from this, the calorie consumption can be determined, provided the calorie content of each quarter sandwich is known. Therefore the sandwiches have to be most carefully prepared, with each of the constituents being weighed as accurately as possible. A selection of four different sandwiches is the usual number presented but there is no limit in principle to the variety of possible choices offered. We have successfully applied this appoach in a study of the anorectic affects of d-Amp (Silverstone and Stunkard, 1968).

(d) *Bite Indicating Telemetering Eatometer (BITE)*. The BITE apparatus devised by Moon (1979) records the rate and frequency at which a subject places food in his mouth using implements (spoon and fork) attached to handles which contain a miniaturized telemetering system. Mouth contact permits a sub-threshold 2 micro-ampere DC current to pass from the utensil to the handle; this produces a radio signal transmitted by a battery-powered radio within the utensil handle. Using appropriate electronic filters and receiver channels, a continuous record can be obtained of all the utensil-to-mouth contacts over a set period. And it is possible, using a multi-channel receiver system recording signals from a number of utensils at once, to monitor the feeding behaviour of several subjects at the same time.

The value of such measures are enhanced when the food to be eaten is placed on a weighing cell; from this a continuous measure of total food intake over the same time period can be obtained. Thus far, no drug studies have been undertaken using these novel electro-mechanical methods. While they might allow an accurate representation to be made of the detailed microstructure of eating, such as the frequency of bites, and the rate of calorie consumption at a set meal, they do not allow more extended observations, nor can they furnish information about food choice.

(e) *Automated Food Dispenser*. In order to avoid the limitations of the approaches described above, yet allowing continuous automatic recording of a subject's intake of solid food over a longer time course, while at the same time allowing for an element of choice in the foods eaten, we devised an automated food dispenser (AFD) which was adapted from a commercially available cold snacks dispenser (Silverstone *et al.*, 1980), Fig. 3.

It is a four-channel refrigerated food dispenser, which is connected to a pen recorder so that every time the subject takes an aliquot of food, the action is recorded on continuously moving paper. This provides a record of the pattern of food intake over time. The longest period over which we have used the apparatus for drug studies is 8 h, but it has been used for other purposes as the sole source of food for subjects over several days (Durrant and Wloch, 1979). The AFD not only provides a record of the quantity of intake, it also discriminates between the choice of food made by the subject each time he or she eats. As there are four channels, each can be loaded with a different food. An important requirement is that the quantity of food in each slot should be relatively small; individually wrapped quarter-sandwiches with the crust removed are ideal. In addition, the portions of food used in any channel must be of a consistent size, weight and calorie content. As long as this is done, a wide variety of foods can be employed. Among foods which we have successfully used in this apparatus have been sandwiches, chocolate wafer biscuits, portions of yoghurt and segments of tangerine. Durrant (personal communication) has greatly extended the range of possible foods. Subjects are in-

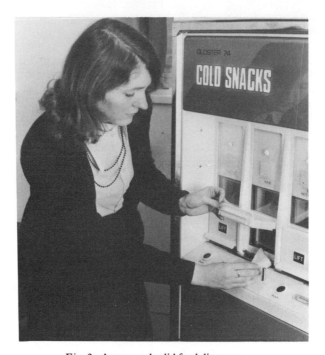

*Fig. 3.* Automated solid food dispenser.

structed to eat as many or as few food aliquots as they like. The only proviso is that they should finish eating one aliquot before pressing the button for another.

In standardization procedures, we have shown this technique of measurement of food intake to be reliable in terms of test–retest reliability, and we have also shown that feeding behaviour measured in this way is highly sensitive to drug effects (Silverstone *et al.*, 1980; Kyriakides and Silverstone, 1979).

## C. Conclusion

For the investigation of the effects of drugs on food intake over a longer-term such as obtains in most clinical trials, indirect measures of food intake such as the diet diary are the most appropriate. Relying entirely on body weight changes to reflect food intake is not justifiable, and attempts to make more accurate measurements are usually impracticable. When diet diaries are being kept in the context of a clinical trial, it is important for patients to receive training in how to use them, particularly when it comes to estimation of portion size.

For shorter-term studies of the effects of single doses of drugs on rate of eating and total intake, undertaken in a laboratory setting, the automated food dispenser appears to be the best of the methods currently available. For more detailed analysis of the microstructure of feeding behaviour, video-tape recording of subjects observed while eating is reliable but time consuming. In the future, recording systems such as that used in the BITE apparatus may provide measures which are as reliable as those obtainable from video-tape analysis, but which are less time-consuming to collect.

# REFERENCES

Aitken, R. C. B. (1969). Measurement of feelings using visual analogue scales. *Proc. Soc. Med.* **62**, 989–993.

Blundell, J. E., Latham, C. J., Moniz, E., McArthur, R. A. and Rogers, P. J. (1979). Structural analysis of the actions of amphetamine and fenfluramine on food intake and feeding behaviour in animals and man. *Curr. Med. Res. Opin.* **6** (Suppl. 1), 34–54.

Durrant, M. and Royston, P. (1979). Short-term effects of energy density on salivation, hunger and appetite in obese subjects. *Int. J. Obes.* **3**, 335-347.

Durrant, M. and Wloch, R. (1978). The effect of palatability on energy intake in two obese women. *Proc. Nut. Soc.* **38**, 37a.

Gagnon, M. A. and Tetreault, L. (1975). Human pharmacology of anorexigens—validity of an appetite questionnaire. *Union. Med. Can.* **104**, 922–929.

Hashim, S. A. and Van Italie, E. (1964). An automatically monitored food dispensing apparatus for the study of food intake in man. *Fed. Proc.* **23** (Pt. 1, No. 1), 82.

Jordan, H. A., Weiland, W. F., Zebley, S. P., Stellar, E. and Stunkard, A. J. (1966). Direct measurement of food intake in man: a method for the objective study of eating behaviour. *Psychosom. Med.* **28**, 836–842.

Kyriakides, M. and Silverstone, T. (1979). A double-blind comparison of fenfluramine and dextroamphetamine on feeding behaviour in man. *Curr. Med. Res. Opin.* **6** (Suppl. 1), 180–187.

Maxwell, C. (1978). Sensitivity and accuracy of the visual analogue scale: a psychophysical classroom experiment. *Brit. J. Clin. Pharmacol.* **6**, 15–24.

Monello, L. F., Seltzer, C. C. and Mayer, J. (1965). Hunger and satiety sensations in men, women, boys and girls. *Ann. N. Y. Acad. Sci.* **131**, 592–602.

Moon, R. D. (1979). Monitoring human eating patterns during the ingestion of non-liquid foods. *Int. J. Obesity* **3**, 281–288.

Pavlov, I. P. (1928). Lectures on Conditional Reflexes. Twenty-five Years of Objective Study of the Higher Nervous Activity (Behaviour) of Animals. Vol. 1. (Trans. and ed. W. H. Guatt (London)), Lawrence and Wishart.

Price, J. M. and Grinker, J. (1973). Effects of degree of obesity, food deprivation and palatability on eating behaviour of humans. *J. Comp. Physiol. Psychol.* **85**, 265–271.

Pudel, V. (1976). Experimental feeding in man. *In* "Appetite and Food Intake" (T. Silverstone, ed.), Abakon, Berlin.

Robinson, R. G., McHugh, P. R. and Folstein, M. F. (1975). Measurement of appetite disturbances in psychiatric disorders. *J. Psychiat. Res.* **12**, 59–68.

Schachter, S. (1971). Some extraordinary facts about obese humans and rats. *Amer. Psychologist* **26**, 129–144.

Silverstone, T. and Fincham, J. (1978). Experimental techniques for the measurement of hunger and food intake in man for use in the evaluation of anorectic drugs. *In*

"Central Mechanisms of Anorectic Drugs" (S. Garrattini and R. Samanin, eds) Raven Press, New York.

Silverstone, T., Fincham, J. and Brydon, J. (1980). A new technique for the continuous measurement of food intake in man. *Amer. J. Clin. Nutr.* (in press).

Silverstone, T. and Schuyler, D. (1975). The effect of cyproheptadine on hunger, calorie intake and body weight in man. *Psychopharmacologia* (Berl.) **40**, 335–340.

Silverstone, J. T., Stark, J. E. and Buckle, R. M. (1966). Hunger during total starvation. *Lancet* i, 1343–1344.

Silverstone, T. and Stunkard, A. J. (1968). The anorectic effect of dexamphetamine sulphate. *Brit. J. Pharmacol. Chemother.* **33**, 513–522.

Silverstone, T., Turner, P. and Humpherson, P. L. (1968). Direct measurement of the anorectic activity of diethylpropion. *J. Clin. Pharmacol.* **8**, 172–179.

Stunkard, A. and Kaplan, D. (1977). Eating in public places: a review of reports of direct observation of eating behaviour. *Int. J. Obesity* **1**, 84–101.

Warner, K. E. and Balagura, S. (1975). Intermeal eating patterns of obese and non-obese humans. *J. Comp. Physiol. Psychol.* **89**, 778–783.

Wooley, S. C. and Wooley, O. W. (1973). Salivation to the sight and thought of food: a new measure of appetite. *Psychosomat. Med.* **35**, 136–142.

# 5 □ Clinical Pharmacology of Appetite

T. Silverstone and M. Kyriakides

## I. APPETITE SUPPRESSANT DRUGS

Anorectic, or appetite suppressant drugs, are drugs which suppress the subjective awareness of hunger. They fall into two broad categories: those acting directly on the central nervous system, and those which act primarily on peripheral mechanisms. The centrally acting anorectic drugs can be further subdivided into: (a) those which have, in addition to their hunger-suppressing action, a central stimulant effect; (b) those which have no such stimulant effect. The peripherally acting compounds act via a number of physiological systems, including the gastrointestinal tract and the regulation of carbohydrate metabolism (see Table I).

*Table I*:  Anorectic drugs.

| | |
|---|---|
| (A) Centrally acting: | |
|     (i) With stimulant properties | Amphetamine (Benzedrine) |
| | Dexamphetamine (Dexedrine) |
| | Phenmetrazine (Preludin) |
| | Phentermine (Duromine) |
| | Diethylpropion (Apisate, Tenuate) |
| | Mazindol (Teronac, Sanorex) |
| | Phenylpropanolamine (Hungrex) |
|     (ii) Without stimulant properties | Fenfluramine (Ponderax, Pondomin) |
| | Tiflorex |
| (B) Peripherally acting: | |
|     (i) Bulk agents | Methylcellulose |
|     (ii) Gastrointestinal hormones and analogues | Cholecystokinin and Octapeptide |
| | Phenylalanine |
|     (iii) Drugs affecting carbohydrate metabolism | Glucagon |
| | Phenformin |
| | Metformin |
|     (iv) Chorionic gondatrophin | |

As with many other significant advances in clinical pharmacology, the first indication that a centrally acting drug might affect hunger arose largely by chance. Amphetamine had been introduced by Alles in 1927 as a synthetic (and therefore cheaper) substitute for ephedrine. It was soon found to be a potent central stimulant, and as a result was introduced for the treatment of narcolepsy. Printzmetal and Bloomberg (1935) noted that one of their patients being treated for narcolepsy with amphetamine who was also overweight lost a significant amount of weight while taking the drug. A similar effect was remarked upon by Davidoff and Reifenstein (1937) who suggested that, because of its anorectic properties, amphetamine might be useful clinically in helping obese patients to lose weight. Lesses and Myerson (1938) were quick to act on this suggestion, and administered amphetamine 15 mg/daily (7.5 mg in the morning, 5 mg at noon and 2.5 mg at 1700 h) to 17 obese patients. They were extremely gratified by the results; not only did the majority of their patients lose weight satisfactorily, the drug also increased the patients' sense of well-being.

Shortly afterwards, Printzmetal and Alles (1940) discovered that the dextro-rotatory isomer of amphetamine, dexamphetamine, was a more potent anorectic than the laevo-isomer and dexamphetamine came to supersede the racemic compound. The euphoriant property of amphetamine which Lesses and Myerson had originally enthused over unfortunately led to amphetamine becoming a drug of abuse, and by the 1950s, amphetamine abuse had become a major problem in a number of countries, although abuse was rarely observed in obese patients who had been prescribed the drug by a doctor to help them lose weight.

Phenmetrazine, introduced in the hope of providing a less stimulating alternative to dexamphetamine, was itself soon found to be just as stimulating, and in consequence was also widely taken up as a drug of abuse. In recent years, a number of alternative compounds have been introduced. Although some of these have stimulant properties (diethylpropion, phentermine, mazindol) they possess a much wider therapeutic ratio than amphetamine; that is, for a given anorectic effect, the stimulant and euphoriant effects are much less than is the case with amphetamine. Fenfluramine, in contrast to the stimulant anorectic drugs thus far considered, was noted to have sedative and depressant properties, despite a close structural similarity to amphetamine (see Fig. 1).

## A.  Centrally-acting Anorectic Drugs with Stimulant Properties

(1)  *Amphetamine (Benzedrine, Dexedrine)*
(a)  *Effect on Subjective Hunger*. Bahnsen et al. (1938) were the first to examine experimentally the anorectic action of amphetamine. In a between-subject trial in which 195 Danish office workers participated, 19 out of the 100 subjects who had been given a single dose of amphetamine (20 mg for men and 10 mg for women) reported a reduction in appetite in response to the question "Has your appetite been increased, reduced or as usual?", whereas only one of the 95 who had been given placebo did so. The anorectic effect, when noted, became

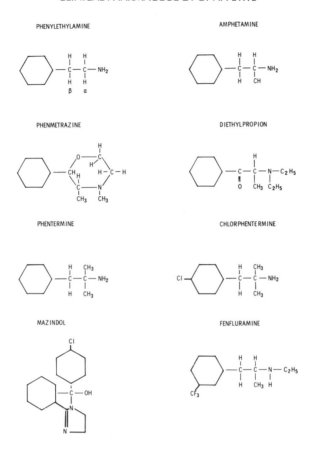

*Fig. 1.* Formulae of anorectic drugs.

apparent within 2 h of ingestion. Jacobsen and Wollstein (1939) obtained similar results in a group of 117 healthy men given 10 mg amphetamine, with appetite reduction being noted more frequently after the active drug than after placebo.

In the course of studies designed primarily to investigate the effect of amphetamine on mood and physical performance, Cuthbertson and Knox (1947) compared 15 mg methamphetamine to placebo in soldiers partaking in a military exercise. Of the 27 soldiers given active drug, only three felt even slightly hungry during a subsequent route march, whereas 11 of the 28 given placebo did. Janowitz and Grossman (1949) remarked that 10 mg dexampheta-mine taken 1 h before lunch abolished all hunger sensations and markedly depressed the desire to eat. Corresponding results were obtained by Smith and Beecher who reported that athletes given amphetamine (14 mg/70 kg) were significantly less likely to tick the word "hunger" when completing an adjective check list concerned with their subjective feelings than when they had been given placebo. Di Mascio and Buie (1964) also noted that a single 10 or 15 mg dose of dexamphetamine lowered appetite in approximately 20% of their male college-student subjects. Hollister (1971) reported that hunger ratings were reduced by dexamphetamine in normal male subjects, but added that in his experience this effect was not striking.

In the studies thus far considered, although amphetamine was significantly more likely than placebo to reduce hunger-related responses in normal subjects completing suitably designed questionnaires, it was usually only a minority of the subjects who appeared to be sensitive to the anorectic effect of the drug. In other studies, no consistent anorectic effect was noted at all (Smith *et al.*, 1963; Bernstein and Grossman, 1956). In contrast to these somewhat inconclusive findings, Gagnon and Elie (1975), in a study comparing the anorectic effect of d-Amp and marijuana found that 7.5 and 15 mg dexamphetamine had a significant anorectic effect, as judged by responses to an appetite questionnaire.

In order to try to obtain a more quantitative assessment of the anorectic properties of dexamphetamine, we used a hunger visual analogue scale (VAS) to determine changes in hunger ratings in a placebo-controlled double-blind cross-over trial of single doses of dexamphetamine in normal male volunteer subjects (Silverstone and Stunkard, 1968). We found that dexamphetamine did have a statistically significant anorectic effect on VAS ratings, and that 10 mg and 15 mg had a greater effect than 5 mg. This finding has been confirmed in subsequent investigations (Kyriakides and Silverstone, 1979; Silverstone *et al.*, submitted for publication; Wells *et al.*, in preparation) (see Fig. 2).

(b) *Effects on Food Intake*. Although it was generally assumed that the weight loss attributable to amphetamine in the treatment of obesity was due to its anorectic action, which in turn led to a reduction in calorie intake, no direct measurements of its effect on food intake were made for some years. Harris *et al.* (1947) were the first to record directly the effects of dexamphetamine on food intake under carefully controlled conditions in obese patients and normal subjects. In the obese patients, dexamphetamine 5–10 mg administered 1 h before meals resulted in a reduction in calorie intake sufficient to account for the weight loss observed. The normal subjects responded similarly but less consistently. The authors' conclusion, which was not entirely justified from the data given, was: "This experiment has clearly shown that amphetamine-induced loss of weight is almost entirely due to anorexia".

Using a standard sandwich meal (see Chapter 4) to measure the effects of dexamphetamine on food intake, we found that 5, 10, 15 and 20 mg dexamphetamine given 2 h before the meal significantly reduced calorie intake as compared to placebo. Hollister (1971) reported that consumption of a standardized chocolate milk shake was reduced in seven out of twelve normal male subjects given dexamphetamine (0.2 mg/kg) 2.5h beforehand, and Gagnon

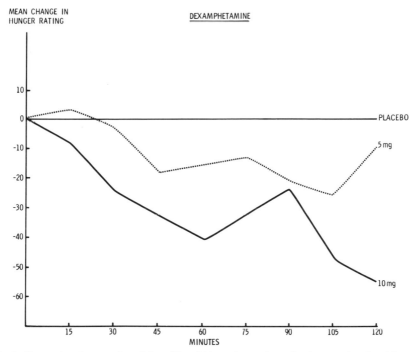

*Fig. 2.* Dose-related anorectic activity of 5 and 10 mg dexamphetamine in normal male subjects. (Silverstone and Stunkard, 1968).

and Tetrault (1975) showed that 5 mg dexamphetamine given 4 h previously significantly reduced the amount eaten during a standard lunch. Blundell *et al.* (1979) observed the effects in six normal male subjects of a single 10 mg oral dose of dexamphetamine on food intake at standard sandwich meals presented 3, 9 and 24 h after drug administration. Following dexamphetamine, there was a 12% reduction in food intake as compared to placebo at the first meal, 9.7% at the second and 9.0% at the third. The greatest suppression was at the first meal, (i.e. 3 h after the drug had been given) and occured when plasma levels of the drug were highest. In a subsequent experiment, in which the meals consisted of bread and cold sliced meats, continuous videotape recordings were made of feeding behaviour. These were analysed in terms of: (a) latency to begin eating, (b) duration of eating, (c) number of mouthfuls, (d) average size of mouthful, (e) inter-mouth interval, (f) rate of chewing and (g) rate of ingestion. Three hours before the meal, 10 mg dexamphetamine administered to 12 subjects significantly reduced total intake. It also increased the latency to begin eating, shortened the duration of the meal, and increased the rate of ingestion.

Using the automated food dispenser described in Chapter 4 to obtain a continuous record of food intake over a 2-h period, beginning 2 h after

administration of 10 mg dexamphetamine to 18 normal female subjects, Kyriakides and Silverstone (1979) found that the drug reduced food intake by
approximately 50% as compared to placebo, and also increased latency to begin
eating. However, in contrast to Blundell *et al.* (1979), we observed a reduction
rather than an increase in the rate of food consumption (see Fig. 3).

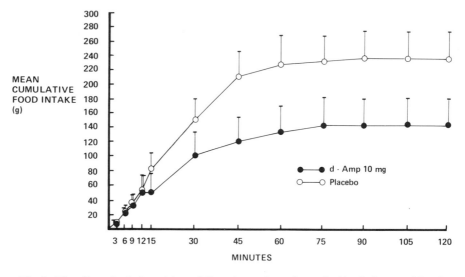

*Fig. 3.* The effect of a single oral dose of 10 mg dexamphetamine on food intake in normal female
subjects during a 2 h recording period which commenced 2 h after the administration of
dexamphetamine (Kyriakides and Silverstone).

(c) *The Relationship of the Effects of Amphetamine on Subjective Hunger Rating
to Its Effect on Food Intake.* In all the studies in which a comparison has been
made of the effects of dexamphetamine on subjective hunger ratings and its
effects on the objective measurement of food intake, a close correspondence
between the two has been observed. Silverstone and Stunkard (1968) found
that the effect on hunger ratings, expressed as a change of rating from the start
of the experiment correlated significantly with its effects on food intake (r =
+0.38, p <0.05). Gagnon and Tetrault (1975) also noted a close relationship
between the subjective anorectic effects of dexamphetamine, as judged by
answers to a hunger questionnaire, and the objective reduction in food intake.
Similarly, we observed that the total amount of food consumed during a 2-h
feeding period, beginning 2 h after the oral administration of 10 mg dexamphetamine, closely paralleled the reduction in VAS hunger ratings obtained at
the start of the feeding period (Kyriakides and Silverstone, 1979). Thus Harris
*et al.* (1947) were right; amphetamine does indeed have a true anorectic
action which leads to a significant reduction in food intake, and this is the most
likely explanation for its efficacy in the treatment of obesity.

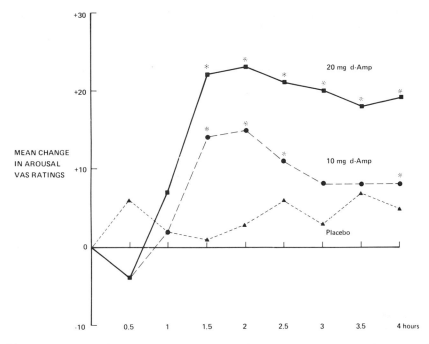

*Fig. 4.* VAS ratings of arousal after single oral doses of 10 and 20 mg dexamphetamine compared to placebo in eight normal male subject. (Silverstone *et al.*, to be published).

## (d) *Stimulant and Euphoriant Effects*

(i) **Subjective effects.** In their study involving Danish office workers, Bahnsen *et al.* (1938) reported that 36% of those who had received amphetamine noticed an increase in alertness, in the sense that they had difficulty in getting off to sleep, whereas only 6.5% of those given placebo did so. Some time later, Lasagna *et al.* (1955) reported that a subcutaneous injection of 20 mg amphetamine administered to 20 normal male subjects caused 12 (60%) to feel definitely more alert. However, in a subsequent study, Goldstein *et al.* (1960) failed to confirm Lasagna's results. It is clear that as far as the stimulant response to amphetamine is concerned, there is wide inter-subject variation. In a further study, less than a third of subjects given 15 mg *d*-amphetamine under double-blind conditions, categorized the drug as stimulant, although this was a larger proportion than that so categorizing placebo (Hurst *et al.*, 1939). However, using a visual analogue scale to quantify the changes in subjective arousal produced by single oral doses of 10 and 20 mg *d*-amphetamine under strictly double-blind conditions, we have found that the drug produces a highly statistically significant dose-related increase in subjective arousal as compared to placebo (Wells and Silverstone, unpublished observations) (see Fig. 4).

**(ii) Effects on sleep.** Amphetamine has been repeatedly found to affect sleep adversely. It particularly reduces the amount of rapid eye movement (REM) sleep, the stage of sleep which is believed to be associated with dreaming (Lewis, 1970). The dextro-rotary (+) isomer of amphetamine has a relatively greater effect on sleep than the laevorotatory (−) isomer (Hartman and Cravens, 1976) and the effects of sleep deprivation are more readily reversed by dexamphetamine than by laevo-amphetamine (Hartman *et al.*, 1977). Such findings indicate a relatively stereo-specific neurochemical mechanism underlying amphetamine-induced sleep disturbance. This mechanism would also appear to be extremely sensitive; plasma concentrations as low as 5 ng/ml can lead to discernable E.E.G. effects (Morselli *et al.*, 1976).

**(iii) Effects on performance.** Psychomotor performance is usually, but not invariably, improved by amphetamine when compared to placebo under double-blind conditions. (See Weis and Laties, 1962; Silverstone and Wells, 1980 for reviews.) Whatever the effect of amphetamine on psychomotor performance tests, subjects frequently think they have done better than they have after taking the drugs; in this sense, amphetamine might be considered to impair judgement (Smith and Beecher, 1964). When the effect of amphetamine on athletic performance was comprehensively examined by Smith and Beecher (1959), they noted a significant improvement in performance among trained athletes in swimming, running, and shot-putting 2 h after amphetamine 14 mg/70 kg. Partly as a result of these findings, the use of stimulant drugs by athletes taking part in competitions was banned.

**(iv) Effects on mood.** In one of the first controlled studies designed to evaluate its euphoriant properties, amphetamine administered subcutaneously to 20 normal volunteer subjects at a dose of 29 mg/70 kg was compared to pentobarbitone, morphine, heroin and placebo (Lasagna *et al.*, 1955). Thirteen of the 20 subjects rated amphetamine as the most pleasant of the drugs they had received, several remarking that they felt particularly "happy" or "enthusiastic". A similar result was obtained in a study involving 239 subjects completing an adjective check list; here too, such words as "happy" and "friendly" were checked more often after amphetamine than after placebo (Cameron *et al.*, 1965). The dextro-rotary isomer was at least twice as potent as laevo-amphetamine in elevating mood in normal subjects (Smith and Davis, 1977). Furthermore, a greater euphoriant action was observed after 20 mg dextroamphetamine than after 10 mg, a finding which we have confirmed using VAS ratings of mood (Wells and Silverstone, unpublished observations) (see Fig. 5).

**(v) Paranoid psychosis.** Amphetamine in high dosage can cause a paranoid psychosis virtually indistinguishable from that occurring in true paranoid schizophrenia, except that amphetamine psychosis resolves completely on withdrawal of the drug (Connell, 1958). This phenomenon has had important implications for theories attempting to explain the pathogenesis of schizophrenia (Crow, 1979).

**(vi) Pharmacokinetics.** The rate of excretion of amphetamine is markedly dependent on urinary pH. At low urinary pH, the drug is significantly more

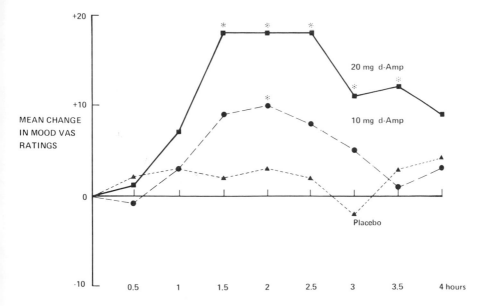

*Fig. 5.* The effect of single doses of 10 and 20 mg dexamphetamine on VAS ratings of mood compared to placebo in eight normal male subjects (Silverstone *et al.*, to be published).

rapidly eliminated than at higher alkaline pH (Beckett *et al.*, 1965). Furthermore, at a low urinary pH, the greater part of the administered amphetamine is excreted unchanged, whereas at a high pH, the aminoalkyl group undergoes oxidative deamination leading to the formation of benzoic acid. Making the urine alkaline by giving sodium bicarbonate, thereby reducing the excretion, and thus increasing the plasma level of amphetamine was found to prolong and enhance its effect on psychomotor function (Smart and Turner, 1966).

Following oral administration of 20 mg dexamphetamine phosphate to six healthy volunteer subjects (four male and two female), plasma levels, measured by a gas–liquid chromatography method, reached a peak concentration of 30–40 ng/ml three to four hours after administration (Morselli *et al.*, 1976). Absorption appeared to follow a biexponential pattern, which may be related to an action of dexamphetamine on the vascular bed of the gastrointestinal tract. Significant clinical effects were noted when the plasma level had reached 20 ng/ml, although E.E.G. changes were observable at a plasma level as low as 5 ng/ml. The plasma half-life was approximately 5 h.

Using a radioimmuno-assay procedure to measure plasma levels of amphetamine following a single oral 30 mg dose in eight depressed patients, Ebert *et al.* (1976) recorded peak plasma levels of 30–60 ng/ml occurring two or three hours after administration; following this, there was a slow decline over the next 24 h. The mean plasma half-life was 20 h (which is longer than the value obtained by Morselli *et al.*, 1976) but there was considerable individual variation. In these patients, there was a significant positive correlation between symptoms of activation experienced subjectively and the measured plasma level.

(f) *Neurochemical Basis for the Central Effects of Amphetamine in Man.* In animals, amphetamine is thought to act mainly by releasing noradrenaline (NA) and dopamine (DA) in the neuronal pathways in which these substances act as neurotransmitters; its stimulant action being particularly related to DA (see Chapter 2). One way of examining whether the same mechanisms underlie the central effects of amphetamine in man is to observe the effects of specific receptor-blocking compounds on amphetamine induced-activity. Using the specific DA receptor-blocking drug pimozide for this purpose, Jonsson (1972) reported that it markedly reduced the subjective stimulant effects of an extremely large (200 mg) dose of dexamphetamine in previously addicted subjects. In keeping with this observation, we have found that pimozide at a dose of 2 and 4 mg attenuates the stimulant effect of more modest (10 mg and 20 mg) doses of dexamphetamine in normal volunteer subjects (Silverstone *et al.*, 1980) (see Fig. 6). Such findings indicate that the stimulant action of amphetamine is likely to be mediated through an action on central dopaminergic pathways.

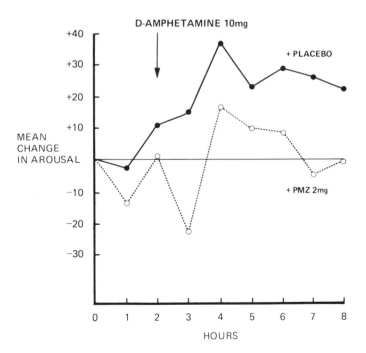

*Fig. 6 (a).* Attenuation by the DA receptor-blocking drug pimozide of the stimulant action of 10 mg d-Amp in normal male subjects

In contrast to its effect on arousal, pimozide had no effect on dexamphetamine-induced anorexia, suggesting that dopaminergic transmission is not involved in mediating the anorectic action of amphetamine. On the other hand thymoxamine, an alpha-noradrenergic receptor-blocking compound did appear to attenuate the anorectic response to amphetamine (Jacobs and Silverstone, in preparation) (see Fig. 7). The implication of this latter finding, if confirmed, is that amphetamine-induced anorexia in man is mediated through an action on central noradrenergic pathways.

## (2) *Phenmetrazine (Preludin)*

Phenmetrazine was introduced in the 1950s in the belief that it was an anorectic drug with less stimulant activity than amphetamine. While it was shown to possess some anorectic effects in normal subjects (Penick and Hinkle, 1964) and obese patients (Briggs *et al.*, 1960), subsequent investigations revealed that contrary to what had been originally thought, the drug did cause significant subjective activation, and elevation of mood (Martin *et al.*, 1971), and it has been widely misused for non-therapeutic purposes. Furthermore, phenmetrazine, when taken in large doses, is as prone as amphetamine to cause a paranoid psychosis indistinguishable from amphetamine psychosis (Evans, 1959).

## (3) *Diethylpropion (Tenuate, Apisate)*

Diethylpropion was another compound which was introduced as an anorectic agent thought to have less stimulant activity than amphetamine. Animal evidence had indicated that, at equipotent anorectic dosage, diethylpropion produced less of an increase in locomotor activity than amphetamine (Hoekenga *et al.*, 1978). Similar findings have been obtained in man, for a given anorectic effect diethylpropion is less stimulating than amphetamine, and has been less a source of drug abuse.

(a) *Effects on Hunger and Food Intake.* The anorectic property of diethylpropion has been confirmed in man, both in normal volunteers and in obese patients. It was shown that 50 mg diethylpropion was approximately equivalent to 10 mg dexamphetamine in lowering hunger VAS ratings, with the maximum effect occurring within 1 h of oral administration (Silverstone, 1975).

Using the long-acting form of diethylpropion (Tenuate Dospan) Silverstone *et al.* (1968) reported that hunger VAS ratings and recorded food intake were significantly reduced by an oral 75 mg dose as compared to placebo in a double-blind controlled study in a group of 18 moderately overweight young women. More recently, we have observed that a single dose of 75 mg diethylpropion (as Tenuate Dospan) significantly reduces food consumption over an 8-h period as measured by the automated solid food dispenser described in Chapter 4 (Kyriakides and Silverstone, unpublished observation) (see Fig. 8).

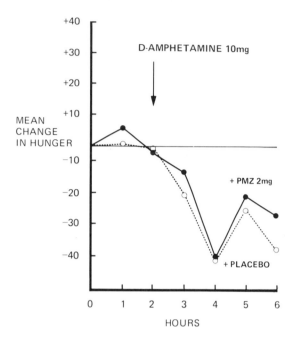

*Fig. 6 (b).* No attenuation by pimozide of the anorectic action of 10 mg d-Amp in normal male subjects.

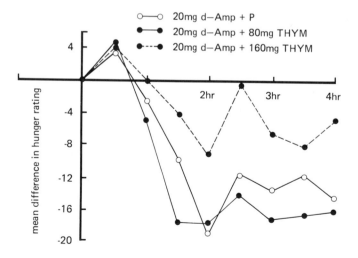

*Fig. 7.* Attenuation by the NA receptor-blocking drug thymoxamine (THYM) of the anorectic activity of 20 mg d-Amp in normal male subjects (Jacobs and Silverstone, in preparation).

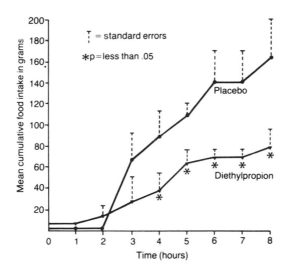

*Fig. 8.* Effect of a single 75 mg dose of the long-acting formulation of diethylpropion (Tenuate Dospan) and placebo on food intake as measured using the automated food dispenser over an 8-h period.

(b) *Stimulant Effects.* As far as the central stimulant effects of diethylpropion are concerned, subjective rating scales revealed that 50 mg led to a non-significant increase in ratings of alertness in normal subjects (Johnsson *et al.*, 1965). Similar results were obtained in moderately obese young women given 75 mg of the long-acting preparation of diethylpropion in whom an increase in ratings of restlessness was found (Silverstone *et al.*, 1968).

Employing the more objective measure of critical flicker fusion, a significant stimulant effect has been observed in two double-blind placebo controlled studies (Sjoberg and Jonsson, 1967; Smart *et al.*, 1967). Furthermore, when the effects of 50 mg diethylpropion, given 1–1.5 h before lights out, on E.E.G. recordings taken during sleep were analysed in four normal volunteer subjects, the drug led to more frequent awakenings, although there was no delay in getting off to sleep (Oswald *et al.*, 1968). If the drug was given during the day, no such E.E.G. effects were seen, probably because of the drug's short half-life, (Lewis *et al.*, 1971).

In contrast to laboratory evidence indicating a stimulant activity in normal volunteer subjects, in a more clinical setting, an evening dose of 25 mg diethylpropion did not lead to any serious deterioration in the sleep of a group of 14 obese patients (Silverstone and Cleary, 1967). Furthermore, although it may have some stimulant properties, the abuse potential of diethylpropion appears to be less than that of amphetamine and phenmetrazine. For example, subjects with a history of amphetamine abuse rated the drug as less desirable than amphetamine (Jasinski, 1974), and the frequency of diethylpropion abuse reported in the Drug Abuse Warning Network set up in the United States compared to the number of prescriptions issued, suggests a relatively low abuse potential (Hoekenga *et al.*, 1978). Nevertheless, when it is abused, diethylpropion can, like amphetamine, lead to the development of a paranoid psychosis.

(c) *Pharmacokinetics.* The pharmacokinetics of diethylpropion are complex, and it has a number of metabolites with varying pharmacological activities (Beckett, 1979). As with amphetamine, excretion is markedly affected by the pH of the urine; excretion is much more rapid at low urinary pH. Under these conditions, the half-life of the parent compound and its active metabolites is some 4–5 h.

### (4) *Phentermine (Duramin)*

Phentermine is yet another phenylethylamine analogue with pronounced anorectic properties, but with less stimulant activity than amphetamine. In six moderately overweight subjects, single doses of 15 and 30 mg phentermine, as the resinate, administered at 0800 h under double-blind conditions led to a significant dose-related reduction in calorie intake at standard sandwich meals presented at 1300 h and 1800 h, as compared to placebo during the day of administration, and the 30 mg dose led to a significant lowering of hunger VAS ratings (Silverstone, 1972). There was a significant correlation found within the subjects between their hunger ratings and food intake on the experimental days. In clinical trials, phentermine would appear to be less stimulating than dexamphetamine, although equally effective as an anorectic (Seaton *et al.*, 1964). Only small effects on the sleeping E.E.G. were noted in normal volunteers after 30 mg phentermine was given the same afternoon (Morselli *et al.*, 1978). As with the other phenylethylamine derivatives thus far considered, the rate of excretion of phentermine is sensitive to changes in urinary pH, excretion being faster at low pH (Beckett and Brookes, 1971). Following oral administration of 12.45 mg phentermine, the elimination half-life was found to be 7–8 h, with the greater part of the dose being excreted unchanged. Comparing the pharmacokinetics of single 30 mg doses of the free salt with the resinate, Morselli *et al.* (1978) reported a peak plasma level of 172 ng/ml eight–nine hours after the resinate.

### (5) *Mazindol (Teronac, Sanorex)*

Although of quite different chemical structure, its pharmacological properties appear similar to those of some of the stimulant anorectic phenylethylamines (Chapter 2).

Surprisingly, in the light of previous animal evidence, mazindol 1 mg daily was reported to have no significant effect on subjective appetite ratings in a group of normal volunteer subjects (Holmstrand and Jonsson, 1975). However in contrast to this finding, a single 1 mg dose of mazindol was noted to reduce calorie intake significantly, as compared to placebo, in normal subjects over an 8-h period (Silverstone and Kyriakides, unpublished observations).

Clinically, it has been found to reduce subjective awareness of hunger and to cause greater weight loss than placebo in a double-blind trial (Haugen, 1975). However, both the anorectic effect and its duration of action may be less than that seen with other available anorectic drugs (Smith, 1975). It has little in the way of stimulant effects as evaluated by critical flicker fusion measures (Hedges, 1972). In a group of prisoners who had previously abused amphetamine, the stimulant and euphoriant effects experienced after a 2 mg dose of mazindol were minimal, and in the opinion of the participating subjects, hardly at all reminiscent of amphetamine (Gottestam and Gunne, 1972).

(6)  *Phenylpropanolamine (Hungrex)*
Phenylpropanolamine (also known as norephedrine or propadrine) is a beta-hydroxylated phenylethylamine derivative which was noted to decrease feeding in rats without increasing locomotion. It also has strong vasoconstrictor and weak bronchodilator effects (see Hoebel, 1977 for review). In 48 normal volunteer subjects, a single oral 25 mg dose of phenylpropanolamine administered at 1200 h led to a significant reduction of intake of liquid nutrient from a hidden reservoir (see Chapter 4) as compared to placebo (Hoebel et al., 1975). When taken at a dose of 25 mg three times daily for two weeks, in a placebo controlled cross-over trial in 70 volunteer subjects desirous of losing weight, phenylpropanolamine caused significantly greater weight loss than placebo (Hoebel et al., 1975); and in a between-patient clinical trial involving 77 obese patients on a 1200 calorie diet, a phenylpropanolamine–caffeine combination led to a greater weight loss than placebo during the four-week trial period (Griboff et al., 1975). This drug is not without risk: phenylpropanolamine-induced renal impairment has been described (Bennett, 1979).

## (B)  Non-stimulant Centrally Acting Anorectic Drugs

(1)  *Fenfluramine (Ponderax, Pondomin)*
Fenfluramine, although chemically a phenylethylamine derivative like most of the stimulant anorectic drugs considered in the preceding section, has a markedly different spectrum of pharmacological activity (see Chapter 2). In particular, its anorectic action appears to be mediated through serotonergic rather than catecholaminergic pathways in the brain, and it possesses no central stimulant properties. Furthermore, in addition to a central action, fenfluramine has an effect on muscle glucose uptake mechanisms which may be of some relevance to its efficacy in the treatment of obesity (see Chapter 6).

(a)  *Effect on Subjective Hunger.*  In a double-blind placebo controlled study in 16 normal subjects (8 male, 8 female), hunger VAS ratings were reduced in a dose-related manner following administration of fenfluramine in single doses of 20, 40 and 80 mg (Silverstone et al., 1975). The highest dose produced the greatest anorectic effect which persisted for 8 h, and which was more marked in the female subjects than in the male. No difference in anorectic activity could be detected between the 20 and the 40 mg doses (see Fig. 9). The degree

MEAN HUNGER RATING - WOMEN

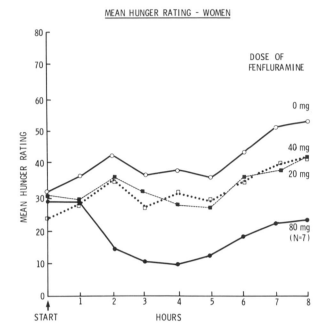

*Fig. 9.* Dose-related anorectic activity of single doses of fenfluramine in normal subjects.

of anorexia observed with each dose closely paralleled the plasma level reached, with the highest mean plasma level (80 ng/ml) occurring in the female subjects 4 h after administration of 80 mg fenfluramine. A similar dose-related effect of fenfluramine on hunger ratings was observed in a more recent study (Kyriakides and Silverstone, 1979). Holmstrand and Jonsson (1975) have also reported a reduction in subjective appetite ratings in sixteen normal subjects given fenfluramine.

Using the salivary response to the sight of palatable food as a measure of hunger (see Chapter 4), Wooley *et al.* (1979) found that 40 mg fenfluramine administered 1 h prior to the ingestion of a liquid "pre-load" enhanced the suppressant effect that this pre-load had on the salivary response to the sight of palatable food 1 h later. Although the authors referred to their findings as denoting appetite suppression, a direct peripheral action on the salivary glands cannot be ruled out, particularly as dry mouth has been a frequently observed side-effect in clinical trials (Pinder *et al.*, 1975).

(b) *Effect on Food Intake.* Pudel (1976) reported that fenfluramine reduced the intake in liquid nutrient obtained through a straw from a hidden reservoir (see Chapter 4). Under controlled conditions in normal volunteer subjects, we have observed a dose-related reduction in calorie intake following single doses of 40, 60 and 80 mg fenfluramine in a placebo-controlled study in which

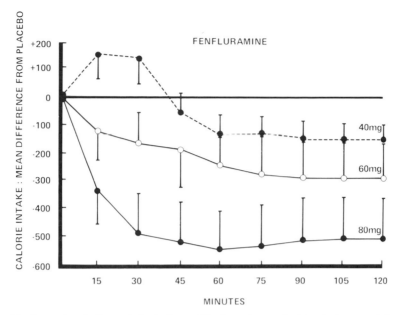

*Fig. 10.* Dose-related effects of single doses of fenfluramine on food intake in normal female subjects.

eighteen normal female subjects participated (Kyriakides and Silverstone, in preparation) (see Fig. 10). The subjects who had been fasting for 8–9 h were given the active drug, or placebo at 1700 h and were allowed access to the automated solid food dispenser 2 h later, that is from 1900 h to 2100 h. There was a similar dose-related pattern observed in the plasma levels of fenfluramine.

In terms of the drug's effect on feeding, we could detect no difference between 60 mg fenfluramine and 10 mg dexamphetamine (Kyriakides and Silverstone, 1979) (see Fig. 11). Both increased the latency to start feeding, and both slowed the rate of eating; the total reduction in calorie intake was also very similar. Blundell *et al.* (1979) reported that 80 mg fenfluramine administered at 0900 h to six male subjects after an overnight fast led to a significant reduction in food intake, as compared to placebo at standard sandwich meals presented 3, 9 and 24 h after the drug had been taken. In a subsequent experiment, these authors carried out detailed analysis of observed feeding behaviour recorded on video tape. Fenfluramine led to the subjects chewing their food for a longer period, thus slowing the "local eating rate". The overall calorie intake and the overall eating rate were also reduced; the subjects consuming an average 173 g in 12.62 min (13.7 g/min) after 60 mg fenfluramine, compared to rate of 237 g in 13.89 min (16.9/min) after placebo. In contrast to our finding that the effects of 60 mg fenfluramine on feeding were indistinguishable from 10 mg dexamphetamine (Kyriakides and Silverstone,

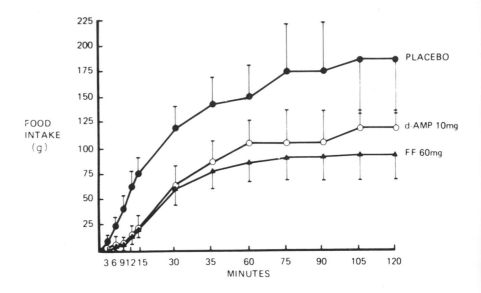

*Fig. 11.* Comparison of dexamphetamine 10 mg and fenfluramine 60 mg on food intake in normal female subjects.

1979), Blundell *et al.* (1979) observed that dexamphetamine led to an *increase* in the "local" eating rate but no change in the overall rate of eating.

(c) *Other Central Effects.* In contrast to the stimulant effects observed with amphetamine, fenfluramine is more likely to lead to drowsiness. This has been observed in normal subjects (Silverstone *et al.*, 1974; Holmstrand and Jonsson, 1975) and in obese patients (Pinder *et al.*, 1975). Again in contrast to amphetamine, mood tends to be depressed rather than elevated, especially after stopping the drug abruptly. This too has been reported in normal subjects (Holmstrand and Jonsson, 1975) and in obese patients both during (Innes *et al.*, 1977) and after stopping drug treatment (Oswald *et al.*, 1971). Amphetamine addicts consistently recognize a qualitative difference between fenfluramine and amphetamine; fenfluramine does not possess the same euphoriant property, and is regarded by these subjects as being much less desirable (Gottestam and Gunne, 1972; Griffith *et al.*, 1975). E.E.G. changes due to fenfluramine are also sharply distinguishable from those of amphetamine, being more like those observed after amylobarbitone (Fink *et al.*, 1971). Psychometric testing using the critical flicker frequency revealed that single 20 and 40 mg doses of fenfluramine had no effect in normal volunteer subjects (Hill and Turner, 1967) but did counter the rise in critical flicker frequency induced by dexamphetamine (Turner, 1971). As far as neurochemical mechanisms are concerned, the finding in man that the level of

5-hydroxyindolacetic acid (the metabolite of 5-hydroxytryptamine) in the cerebrospinal fluid is reduced by fenfluramine is consistent with the view that the central actions of fenfluramine are mediated through serotonergic pathways in the brain (Shoulson and Chase, 1975).

(d) *Pharmacokinetics*. Fenfluramine is readily absorbed from the gastrointestinal tract and tends to accumulate in the tissues owing to its high lipid solubility; this leads to relatively low plasma levels. After multiple dosage, plasma levels build up slowly with a steady state being reached after three or four days (Pinder *et al.*, 1975). There is wide inter-individual variation in the plasma half-life with a range of 14–30 h having been reported (mean value 20 h). Fenfluramine is metabolized by demethylation to the active metabolite norfenfluramine (Beckett, 1979). Under conditions of an acidic urine, more drug and metabolites were recovered unchanged, with the elimination half-life falling to 11 h for both fenfluramine and norfenfluramine.

Turner (1979) showed that fenfluramine had a marked influence on glucose uptake in isolated human muscle preparations *in vitro*, an effect which was blocked by methysergide (a 5-hydroxytryptamine receptor antagonist). He suggested that the efficacy of fenfluramine in obesity could be at least partly explained on the basis of a peripheral action; a view with which Garrow's evidence appeared to be incompatible. Garrow had noted that, in hospital patients on a carefully monitored 800 kcal diet, the addition of fenfluramine led to no additional weight loss (Garrow *et al.*, 1972).

## (2) *Tiflorex*

The slow-release form of this derivative of fenfluramine given as a single 20 mg dose in a double-blind study was shown to possess a significant anorectic effect in man as measured both by subjective hunger VAS ratings and by food intake measurements (Silverstone *et al.*, 1979); the time of maximal subjective activity coincided with the time of maximum reduction of food intake. Tiflorex at this dose appeared to be without any significant effect on the sleep E.E.G. (Morselli *et al.*, 1978).

## C. Peripherally Acting Anorectic Drugs

### (1) *Drugs Affecting Carbohydrate Metabolism*

(a) *Diguanides*. While the diguanide compounds metformin and phenformin alter carbohydrate metabolism in obese diabetic patients, and appear to help such patients lose weight, their value in non-diabetic obesity is less clear (see Chapter 6). Current opinion would indicate that these drugs do not have a primary anorectic effect and they are consequently relatively ineffective in the treatment of uncomplicated obesity (Roginsky and Barnett, 1966; Hart and Cohen, 1970). In any case, metformin was found to be clearly less effective than fenfluramine in promoting weight loss; the likely inference being that it is equally less effective in reducing hunger. Even where a significant weight loss has been produced by diguanides, this was not thought to be attributable to a primary anorectic action (Munro *et al.*, 1969).

(b) *Glucagon.* There have been very few studies of the effect of glucagon on hunger and even fewer on its potential use as a therapeutic agent in obesity. In one experiment of four healthy male volunteers, 1 mg glucagon by intra-muscular injection caused previously hungry subjects to rate themselves as "not hungry" 2 h later (Penick and Hinkle, 1963). The anorectic effect was greater than that following oral phenmetrazine 25 mg, although in the case of phenmetrazine, the rating was made only 1 h after ingestion; this may have been too soon to obtain a significant effect. The anorectic action of glucagon might be related to its inhibitory effect on the motor activity of the fasting stomach, or it might be centrally mediated (Penick *et al.*, 1963) (see Chapter 1 for further discussion on this point).

(c) *Fenfluramine.* As already mentioned, in addition to its central action fenfluramine has an effect on peripheral glucose uptake mechanisms, and this is thought to be of clinical significance by some authorities (Turner, 1978).

## (2) *Bulk Agents*

The idea of filling up the stomach with an inert, non-digestible bulk agent has a refreshing simplicity about it. Unfortunately, trials of methylcellulose have failed to indicate that it helps obese patients lose weight by causing them to eat less (Duncan *et al.*, 1960; Hossain and Campbell, 1975). More direct examina-tion of the anorectic potency of methylcellulose in doses up to 3.375 g (nine tablets) using the VAS did not reveal any hunger-reducing activity whatsoever (Silverstone, 1968). Similar negative results were obtained using a personal-ized hunger rating scale (Durrant and Royston, 1979).

## (3) *Cholecystokinin*

Intravenous infusion of the gastrointestinal hormone cholecystokin (CCK) has been shown to suppress food intake in a number of species and to inhibit sham feeding in rats and monkeys, probably via an action on gastric emptying (see Chapter 1). In man, the effects of CCK on food intake have been less consistent. In one study, rapid intravenous infusion decreased feeding, as measured by consumption of liquid nutrient, while at a slower rate of infusion, CCK increased consumption (Sturdevant and Goetz, 1976). In a more recent study, at a dose within the physiological range, CCK led to a significant reduction of food intake, accompanied by an acceleration of the satiety process (Kissileff *et al.*, 1979). Subjective ratings of satiety also showed the substance to have a satiety effect particularly in the presence of food stimuli (Stacher *et al.*, 1979). In keeping with these reports, phenylalanine, an amino acid which is a potent stimulus for the release of endogenous CCK, has been found to increase satiety VAS ratings in normal subjects as compared to isocaloric lactose placebo (Fincham *et al.*, 1977).

(4) *Chorionic Gonadotrophin*

Chorionic gonadotrophin (HCG) was introduced for the treatment of obesity some 25 years ago by Simeons (1954), who remarked on the loss of appetite it produced, thereby allowing obese patients receiving daily injections of 120 iu to tolerate a 500 kcal diet with equanimity. Unfortunately, subsequent double-blind trials failed to show any superiority of HCG over saline injections (Carne, 1961; Frank, 1964), and in some cases, appetite was reported to have increased rather than decreased. However, another double-blind study revealed a distinct advantage for HCT in terms of anorexia, weight loss and sense of well-being (Asher and Harper, 1973) but this finding was in turn subsequently challenged (Hirsch and Van Itallie, 1973). Whatever the relative anorectic potency of HCG, its mode of action remains obscure.

## II. APPETITE STIMULATING DRUGS

Drugs which stimulate hunger and food intake are sometimes referred to as orexigenic drugs. By stimulating hunger and food intake, these compounds can promote weight gain, and have been used clinically in the management of anorexic states (see Chapter 7).

## A. Centrally Acting Orexigenic Drugs

(1) *Cyproheptadine (Periactin)*

Cyproheptadine is an antihistamine compound which also possesses potent antiserotonergic properties. When administered to asthmatic children, it was noted to promote weight gain. And in a subsequent controlled trial, weight gain attributable to cyproheptadine was found to be significantly greater than that associated with chlorampheniramine, a compound with an equivalent antihistamine effect (Lavenstein *et al.*, 1962). As there was no evidence that cyproheptadine altered metabolism or caused water retention; the weight gain observed was thought to be due to an increased calorie intake, which itself was secondary to a stimulation of appetite. Similar observations have been made in other groups of children (Bergen, 1964), and in adults (Drash *et al.*, 1966; Valiente *et al.*, 1967; Noble, 1969; General Practitioners Research Group, 1970). Cyproheptadine has also been reported to promote weight gain in anorexia nervosa (see Chapter 7).

Although in these earlier reports, comments were made regarding the appetite-stimulating properties of cyproheptadine, in only two studies was any attempt made to quantify this effect, and then only in relatively crude terms such as "appetite restored to normal", "improved" or "no effect" (General Practitioner Research Group, 1970); or "very poor" to "excellent" (Noble, 1969).

This appetite-stimulating property of cyproheptadine, a drug with serotonergic receptor-blocking action, is obviously relevant to the hypothesis that central serotonergic mechanisms play an important role in the regulation of food intake (Blundell, 1977). In a carefully controlled, double-blind study of the effects of 4 mg cyproheptadine administered orally three times daily over a period of three months on appetite ratings and body weight in a group of 26 underweight, but otherwise normal adults was compared to the effects of placebo taken by a control group of 25 subjects (Pawlowski, 1975). Appetite was rated at every visit on a four-point scale (0 = nausea; 1 = none; 2 = good; 3 = excellent). Both appetite ratings and weight gain were greater in the cyproheptadine group, although the differences only reached statistical significance at the sixth to twelfth week with respect to appetite, and at the sixth week with respect to body weight. Cyproheptadine had no detectable effect on thyroid function. In a similar type of investigation, we took the question a stage further by asking our underweight, but otherwise normal subjects, to complete a daily diet diary as well as completing daily hunger ratings (Silverstone and Schuyler, 1975). Furthermore, we used a cross-over trial design, so that each subject had 1 month on cyproheptadine and 1 month on placebo under double-blind conditions. All nine subjects who completed the trial gained significantly more weight on cyproheptadine than on placebo; the mean values being a gain of 1.98 kg ($\pm$0.28) on cyproheptadine and 0.21 kg ($\pm$0.32) on placebo. The daily calorie intake, calculated from the diet diaries, was also somewhat greater during the period on cyproheptadine; 2905 kcal on active drug compared to 2633 kcal on placebo. Finally, evening hunger ratings were higher when the subjects were on cyproheptadine than when they were on placebo. But in contrast to Paulowski (1975) who reported no side-effects attributable to cyproheptadine, eight of our nine subjects complained of drowsiness on the active drug but not on placebo, and a further three subjects withdrew from the trial because of this symptom.

The effects of cyproheptadine on calorie intake were measured directly in two subjects by Saleh (1979) using an automated liquid nutrient dispenser (see Chapter 4). Calorie intake and body weight were significantly increased by cyproheptadine as compared to placebo. The drug had no appreciable effect on energy output.

The findings of all these studies are consistent with the view that the weight gain observed in patients receiving cyproheptadine is due to a true appetite-stimulating action of the drug; it has even been referred to as the first clinically proven appetite stimulant (Lancet, 1978). Furthermore, such evidence is compatible with Blundell's (1975) hypothesis that serotonergic mechanisms are involved in the mediation of hunger and satiety in man.

## (2) Methysergide (Deseril, Sansert)

This compound, which also has pronounced serotonergic receptor-blocking properties, has been reported to cause weight gain in patients receiving it in the course of treatment for migraine (Graham, 1967). In a preliminary pilot study, we have observed that a single oral dose of 1 mg leads to an increase in hunger VAS ratings in normal subjects (Kyriakides and Silverstone, unpublished observations).

(3) *Chlorpromazine and Related Compounds*

Chlorpromazine (Largactil, Thorazine) was the first of the phenothiazine group of compounds to be introduced into psychiatric practice for the treatment of schizophrenia. It was seen to cause weight gain in patients receiving it. Subsequently, other members of this class of drugs have been found to have a similar effect on body weight, although chlorpromazine appeared to be more prone to produce it than the others (Klein and Davis, 1969). Similar weight gain has been reported to follow administration of depot phenothiazines and thioxanthine analogues (Andisen, 1964; Johnson and Breen, 1979).

A number of possible explanations for this effect have been put forward, including fluid retention and/or decreased energy output due to oversedation, but there is little evidence to support such ideas. Patients who gain weight while on these drugs frequently volunteer that they experience intense hunger, and insist that their voracious hunger causes them to overeat and thus gain weight. In a study designed to evaluate disturbances of appetite seen in psychiatric disorders, Robinson *et al.* (1975) observed that patients who were receiving large ($>1.5$ g/day) doses of chlorpromazine had much higher hunger VAS ratings than similar patients on lower doses. Furthermore, the increase in hunger ratings seen in the high-dose patients was accompanied by a marked gain in weight not observed in the others.

As similar changes in body weight are not seen in patients receiving other antipsychotic drugs, such as pimozide, which have a much more specific DA receptor-blocking action than the phenothiazines, it is unlikely that the appetite-stimulating effect of chlorpromazine is due to an action on DA pathways. Rather, it is probable that it is due to one or more of its other pharmacological properties which include antihistaminic and antiserotonergic actions. In keeping with the possibility that its orexigenic effect is related to an action on a central serotonergic mechanism is the report that chlorpromazine-induced weight gain can be ameliorated by the anorectic drug, fenfluramine, a compound which acts by activating serotonergic pathways (Jensen and Kirk, 1972).

(4) *Amitriptyline and Related Compounds*

It is not surprising that an increase in weight is observed following successful drug treatment of depressive illness for loss of appetite and body weight are prominent clinical features of the illness, and clinical improvement is accompanied by an associated improvement of appetite and a consequent gain in weight. However, a number of antidepressant compounds appear to promote a gain in weight over and above that to be expected on the basis of a general overall improvement in clinical state (Kalucy, 1980). Continued medication with amitriptyline (Tryptizol) in patients who had recently recovered from a depressive illness promoted significantly greater weight gain than in a matched control group (Paykel *et al.*, 1973). The patients on amitriptyline complained of an excessive craving for carbohydrates which was not a reflection of any underlying change in glucose tolerance or insulin level. When the amitriptyline was stopped, the craving for carbohydrate disappeared and the excess weight was lost.

A further refutation of the possibility that amitriptyline might be acting on carbohydrate metabolism through an action on insulin secretion was provided by Nakro *et al.* (1977). They could detect no effect on glucose tolerance or insulin levels by amitriptyline in six normal subjects, although two of the six subjects noted definite increase in appetite. It is thus likely that amitriptyline promotes weight gain by increasing appetite through an action on the central neurochemical pathways regulating hunger.

### (5) *Benzodiazepine Derivatives*

In laboratory animals, benzodiazepine compounds such as chlordiazepoxide (Librium) and diazepam (Valium) have been found to promote increased food intake. However, it is uncertain whether this is due to a true orexigenic effect or whether it is the result of changed attitudes to novel or preferred foods (Cooper and Crummy, 1978). In any case, weight gain is rarely observed in patients treated with benzodiazepines in clinical practice (Greenblatt and Shader, 1974).

## B. Peripherally Acting Orexigenic Drugs

### (1) *Insulin*

Insulin has long been known to promote the sensation of hunger. In an investigation carried out shortly after its introduction into clinical practice, Bulateo and Carlson (1924) observed that the administration of insulin by injection was followed by an increase in hunger; however the hunger response did not occur until some 10–60 min after the injection.

Almost 50 years later, using VAS ratings in normal subjects, we confirmed the orexigenic response to insulin (0.15 U/kg) was not immediate, but only occurred after some 30 min delay (Silverstone and Besser, 1971). During the initial period, when blood glucose levels were falling sharply, hunger ratings hardly changed; it was only when the level of blood glucose began to rise that any consistent increase in hunger ratings was observed.

While such a finding is consistent with the "glucostatic" theory of hunger regulation postulated by Mayer (1953), the changes in glucose which we were studying were outside the physiological range. Smaller fluctuations in blood sugar were not found to be accompanied by any increase in hunger (Quaade and Juhl, 1962), and it is unlikely that alteration in blood sugar utilization rates plays any significant role in the regulation of hunger under normal circumstances; it is probably more of an emergency mechanism coming into play only at extreme levels of food deprivation. The clinical application of insulin-induced hunger is discussed in Chapter 7.

### (2) *Lithium*

Weight gain is a well recognized complication of lithium prophylaxis used in the management of recurrent affective disorders. In one group of patients, a gain of at least 5 kg occurred in over 10% of those being studied (Schou *et al.*,

1970), while in another group, the proportion reporting significant weight gain was even higher (Vendsborg *et al.*, 1976). Although one third of the patients in the latter study experienced an increase in appetite, this did not appear to correlate with weight gain; the mean increase in weight among those who felt hungrier was 10.6 kg, a figure which closely resembled the gain of 9.5 kg observed in those who had not noted any increase in hunger. However, there was a close correspondence between increased thirst and weight gain, suggesting that the increase in weight was secondary to an increased consumption of calorie-containing cold drinks taken to assuage thirst. This in turn was probably a consequence of lithium-induced polyuria, a well recognized complication of lithium treatment.

## III. CONCLUSIONS

In this chapter, we have illustrated how centrally acting drugs can influence hunger and feeding behaviour in man in a reproducible and quantifiable manner. The observation that drugs, which in animals act on specific neurochemical pathways (see Chapter 2), can cause predictable and consistent changes in hunger in man implies that the regulation of hunger and food intake in man is under drug-sensitive neurochemical control.

Detailed pharmacological analysis of these drug effects using relatively specific receptor-blocking compounds can throw new light on the neurochemical mechanisms involved in the regulation of hunger and food intake, and help to elucidate the underlying abnormalities in those disease states in which appetite is affected. This in turn should lead to the development of more effective and specific remedies for such clinical conditions.

### REFERENCES

Alles, G. A. (1927). Comparative physiological action of phenylethanol amine. *J. Pharmacol.* **32**, 121–133.

Amdisen, A. (1964). Drug-produced obesity—experience with chlorpromazine, perphenazine and clopenthixol. *Dan. Med. Bull.* **ii**, 18–189.

Asher, W. L. and Harper, H. W. (1973). Effect of human chlorionic gonadotrophin on weight loss, hunger and feeling of wellbeing. *Amer. J. Clin. Nutr.* **26**, 211–218.

Bahnsen, P., Jacobsen, E. and Thesleff, H. (1938). The subjective effect of β-phenylisopropylaminsulfate on normal adults. *Acta. Med. Scan.* **97**, 89–131.

Beckett, A. H. (1979). A comparative study of the pharmacokinetics of fenfluramine, ethylamphetamine, diethylpropion and their metabolites. *Curr. Med. Res. Opin.* **6**, Suppl. 1, 107–117.

Beckett, A. H. and Brookes, L. G. (1971). The metabolism and urinary excretion in man of phentermine, and the influence of N-methyl and p-chloro-substitution. *J. Pharm. Pharmacol.* **23**, 288–294.

Beckett, A. H., Rowland, M. and Turner, P. (1968). Influence of urinary pH in excretion of amphetamine. *Lancet* **i**, 303.

Bennett, W. M. (1979). Hazards of the appetite suppressant phenylpropanolamine. *Lancet* **ii**, 42–43.

Bergen, S. S. (1964). Appetite stimulating properties of cyproheptadine. *Amer. J. Dis. Child.* **108**, 270–272.

Bernstein, L. M. and Grossman, M. I. (1956). An experimental test of the glucostatic theory of regulation of food intake. *J. Clin. Invest.* **35**, 627–633.

Blundell, J. E. (1977). Is there a role for 5HT in feeding? *Int. J. Obesity* **1**, 15–42.

Blundell, J., Latham, C., Moniz, E., McArthur, R. and Rogers, P. (1979). Structural analysis of the actions of amphetamine and fenfluramine on food intake and feeding behaviour in animals and in man. *Curr. Med. Res. Opin.* **6**, Suppl. 1, 34–54.

Blundell, J. E. and Leshem, M. D. (1975). Hypothalamic lesions and drug-induced anorexia. *Postgrad. Med. J.* **51**, Suppl. 1, 45–54.

Briggs, J. H., Newland, P. M. and Bishop, P. M. F. (1960). Phenmetrazine hydrochloride in treatment of obesity. *Brit. Med. J.* **ii**, 911–912.

Bulateo, E. and Carlson, A. J. (1924). Influence of experimental changes in blood sugar levels on gastric hunger contractioans. *Amer. J. Physiol.* **69**, 107–115.

Cameron, J. S., Specht, P. G. and Wendt, G. R. (1965). Effects of amphetamines on moods, emotions and motivation. *J. Psychol.* **61**, 93–121.

Carne, S. (1961). The action of chorionic gonadotrophin in the obese. *Lancet* **ii**, 1282.

Connell, P. H. (1958). Amphetamine psychosis. Maudsley Monograph, Oxford University Press, London.

Cooper, S. J. and Crummy, Y. M. T. (1978). Enhanced choice of familiar food in a food preference test after chlordiazepoxide administration. *Psychopharmacology* **59**, 51–56.

Crow, T. J. (1979). What is wrong with dopaminergic transmission in schizophrenia? *Trends in Neurosciences* **2**, 52–55.

Cuthbertson, D. P. and Knox, J. A. C. (1947). The effects of analytics in the fatigued subject. *J. Physiol.* **106**, 42–58.

Davidoff, E. and Reifenstein, E. C. (1937). Psychopharmacology of chlorphentermine and d-amphetamine. *Clin. Pharmacol. Therap.* **5**, 174–184.

Drash, A., Elliott, J., Langs, H., Lavenstein, A. G. and Cook, R. E. (1966). The effect of cyproheptadine on carbohydrate metabolism. *Clin. Pharmacol. Ther.* **7**, 340–346.

Duncan, L. J. P., Rose, K. and Meiklejohn, A. P. (1960). Phenmetrazine, HCl and methylcellulose in the treatment of 'refractory' obesity. *Lancet* **im**, 1262–1265.

Durrant, M. and Royston, P. (1979). Short term effects of energy density on salivation, hunger and appetite in obese subjects. *Int. J. Obesity* **3**, 335–347.

Ebert, M. H., Van Kammen, D. P. and Murphy, D. L. (1976). Plasma levels of amphetamine and behavioural response. *In* "Pharmacokinetics of Psychoactive Drugs" (L. A. Gottschalk and S. Merlis, eds), pp. 157–169, Spectrum, New York.

Evans, J. (1959). Psychosis and addiction to phenmetrazine. *Lancet* **ii**, 152–155.

Fincham, J., Silverstone, T. and Saha, B. (1977). The effect of *l*-phenylalanine on subjective hunger and satiety in man. Paper presented at 6th International Conference of the Physiology of Food and Water Intake, Paris.

Fink, M., Shapiro, D. M. and Itil, T. M. (1971). E.E.G. profiles of fenfluramine, amobarbital and dextroamphetamine in normal volunteers. *Psychopharmacologia* **22**, 369–383.

Frank, B. W. (1964). The use of chorionic gonadotrophin hormone in the treatment of obesity. *Amer. J. Clin. Nutr.* **14**, 133–136.

Gagnon, M. A. and Elie, R. (1975). Les effets de la marijuana et de la d-amphétamine sur l'appétit, la consommation alimentaire et quelques variables cardio-respiratoires chez l'homme. *Union. Med. Canada* **104**, 914–921.

Gagnon, M. A. and Tétreault, L. (1975). Pharmacologie humaine des anorexigènes— validite d'un questionnaire sur l'appétit. *Union. Med. Canada* **104**, 922–929.

Garrow, J. S., Belton, E. A. and Daniels, A. (1972). A controlled investigation of the 'glycolyptic' action of fenfluramine. *Lancet* ii, 559–561.

General Practice Research Group (1970). A weight promoting drug. *Practitioner* **235**, 101–105.

Goldstein, A., Searle, B. W. and Schinke, R. (1960). Effects of secobarbitol and of d-amphetamine in psychomotor performance of normal subjects. *J. Pharmacol. and Exp. Therap.* **130**, 55.

Gotestam, K. G. and Gunne, L. M. (1972). Subjective effects of two anorexigenic agents fenfluramine and AN 448 in amphetamine dependent subjects. *Brit. J. Addict.* **67**, 39–44.

Graham, J. R. (1967). Current therapeutics—methysergide. *Practitioner* **198**, 302–311.

Greenblatt, D. J. and Shader, R. I. (1974). "Benzodiazepines in Clinical Practice". Raven Press, New York.

Griboff, S. I., Berman, R. and Silverman, H. I. (1975). A double-blind clinical evaluation of a phenylpropanolamine–caffeine–vitamin combination and a placebo in the treatment of exogenous obesity. *Curr. Ther. Res.* **17**, 535–543.

Griffith, J. D., Nutt, J. G. and Jasinski, D. R. (1975). A comparison of fenfluramine and amphetamine in man. *Clin. Pharmacol. Ther.* **18**, 563–570.

Harris, S. C., Ivy, A. C. and Searle, C. M. (1947). The mechanism of amphetamine induced loss of weight. *J. Amer. Med. Ass.* **134**, 1468–1475.

Hart, A. and Cohen, H. (1970). Treatment of obese non-diabetic patients with phenformin—a double-blind cross-over trial. *Brit. Med. J.* i, 22–24.

Hartmann, E. and Cravens, J. (1976). Sleep: effects of d- and l-amphetamine in man and in rat. *Psychopharmacology* **50**, 171–175.

Hartmann, E., Orzack, M. H. and Branconnier, R. (1977). Sleep deprivation deficits and their reversal by d- and l-amphetamine. *Psychopharmacology* **53**, 185–189.

Haugen, H. N. (1975). Double-blind cross-over study of a new appetite suppressant AN 448. *Eur. J. Clin. Pharmacol.* **8**. 71–74.

Hedges, A. (1972). AN 448 on critical flicker frequency and heart rate in man. *S. Afr. Med. J.* **46**, 139.

Hill, R. C. and Turner, P. (1967). Fenfluramine and critical flicker frequency. *J. Pharm. Pharmacol* **19**, 337.

Hirsch, J. and Van Italie, T. B. (1973 ). The treatment of obesity. *Amer. J. Clin. Nutr.* **26**, 1039–1041.

Hoebel, B. G. (1977). The psychopharmacology of feeding. *In* "Handbook of Psychopharmacology" (L. Iversen, S. Snyder and S. Iversen, eds), Vol. 8, 51–127, Raven Press, New York.

Hoebel, B. G., Cooper, J., Kamin, M. C. and Willard, D. (1975). Appetite suppression by phenylpropanolamine in humans. *Obesity Bariatric Med.* **4**, 192–197.

Hoebel, B. G., Krauss, I. K., Cooper, J. and Willard, D. (1975). Body weight decreased in humans by phenylpropanolamine taken before meals. *Obesity Bariatric Med.* **4**, 200–206.

Hoekenga, M. T., O'Dillon, R. H. and Leyland, H. M. (1978). A comprehensive review of diethylpropion hydrochloride. *In* "Central Mechanisms of Anorectic Drugs" (S. Garattini and R. Samanin, eds), pp. 391–404, Raven Press, New York.

Hollister, L. E. (1971). Hunger and appetitite, after single doses of marihuana, alcohol and dextroamphetamine. *Clin. Pharm. Therap.* **12**, 44–49.

Holmstrand, J. and Jonsson, J. (1975). Subjective effects of two anorexigenic agents — fenfluramine and AN 488 in normal subjects. *Postgrad. Med. J.* **51**, 183–186.

Hossain, M. and Campbell, D. B. (1975). Fenfluramine and methyl cellulose in the treatment of obesity: the relationship between plasma drug concentrations and therapeutic efficacy. *Postgrad. Med. J*. **51**, Suppl. 1, 178–182.

Hurst, P. M., Weidner, M. F., Radlow, R. and Ross, S. (1939). Drugs and placebos: drug guessing by naval volunteers. *Psychol. Rep*. **33**, 683–694.

Innes, J. A., Watson, M. L., Ford, M. J., Munro, J. F., Stoddart, M. E. and Campbell, D. B. (1977). Plasma fenfluramine levels, weight loss and side effects. *Brit. Med. J*. **ii**, 1322–1325.

Jacobsen, E. and Wollstein, A. (1939). Studies on the subjective effects of the cephalotropic amines in man. *Acta. Med. Scan*. **100**, 159–187.

Janowitz, H. D. and Grossman, M. I. (1949). Gastro-olfactory thresholds in relation to appetite and hunger sensation. *J. Appl. Physiol*. **2**, 217–222.

Jasinski, D. R. (1974). Effects of diethylpropion and d-amphetamine after subcutaneous and oral administration. *Clin. Pharm. Therap*. **16**, 645–652.

Jensen, P. S. and Kirk, L. (1972). Fenfluramine (Ponderal) in the treatment of adipositas caused by neuroleptics. Paper presented at the Annual Meeting of the Scandinavian Society of Psychopharmacology, Copenhagen.

Johnson, D. and Breen, M. (1979). Weight changes with depot neuroleptics. *Acta. Psychiat. Scan*. **59**, 325–328.

Jonsson, C. O., Sjoberg, L. and Vallbo, S. (1965). Studies in the psychological effects of a new drug (diethylpropion). *Scan. J. Psychol*. **6**, 52–58.

Jonsson, L. E. (1972). Pharmacological blockade of amphetamine: effects in amphetamine dependent subjects. *Eur. J. Clin. Pharm*. **4**, 206–211.

Kalucy, R. S. (1980). Drug induced weight gain. *Drugs* **19**, 268–278.

Kissileff, H. R., Pi-Sunyer, F. X., Thornton, J. and Smith, G. P. (1979). Cholesystokinin-octapeptide (CCK-8) decreases food intake in man. *Amer. J. Clin. Nutr*. **32**, 939–944.

Klein, D. F. and Davis, J. M. (1969). "Diagnosis and Drug Treatment of Psychiatric Disorders". Williams and Wilkins, Baltimore.

Kyriakides, M. and Silverstone, T. (1979). Comparison of the effects of d-amphetamine and fenfluramine on hunger and food intake in man. *Neuropharmacology* **18**, 1007–1008.

Lancet (1978). *Cyroheptadine*. **i**, 362–368.

Lasagna, L., Von Felsinger, J. M. and Beecher, H. K. (1955). Drug induced mood changes in man. Observations on healthy subjects, chronically ill patients and post-addicts. *J. Amer. Med. Ass*. **157**, 1006–1020.

Lavenstein, A. F., Decaney, E. P., Lasagna, L. and Van Metre, T. (1962). Effect of cyroheptadine on asthmatic children: a study of appetite, weight gain and linear growth. *J. Amer. Med. Ass*. **180**, 912–916.

Lesses, M. F. and Myerson, A. (1938). Benzedrine sulphate as an aid to the treatment of obesity. *New Eng. J. Med*. **218**, 119–124.

Lewis, S. A. (1970). Comparative side-effects of some amphetamine derivatives on human sleep. *In* "Amphetamines and Related Compounds" (E. Costa and S. Garattini, eds), pp. 873–888, Raven Press, New York.

Lewis, S. A., Oswald, Z. and Dunleavy, D. C. F. (1971). Chronic studies of fenfluramine and diethylpropion on human sleep. Seminar on Fenfluramine, Nassau.

Martin, W. R., Sloan, J. W., Sapira, J. D. and Jasinski, D. R. (1971). Physiologic, subjective and behavioural effects of amphetamine, methamphetamine, ephedrine, phenmetrazine and methylphenidate in man. *Clin. Pharm. Therap*. **12**, 245–258.

Mayer, J. (1953). Glucostatic mechanism of regulation of food intake. *New Eng. J. Med*. **249**, 13–16.

Morselli, P. L., Placidi, G. F., Maggini, C., Gomeni, R., Guazelli, M., De Listio, G., Standen, S. and Tognoni, G. (1976). An integrated approach for the evaluation of psychotropic drugs in man. *Psychopharmacologia* **46**, 211–217.

Morselli, P. L., Maggini, C., Placidi, G. F., Gomeni, R. and Tognoni, G. (1978). An integrated approach to the clinical pharmacology of anorectic drugs. *In* "Central Mechanisms of Anorectic Drugs" (S. Garattini and R. Samanin, eds), pp. 243–266, Raven Press, New York.

Munro, J. F., MacCuish, A. C., Marshall, A., Wilson, E. and Duncan, L. J. P. (1969). Weight reducing effect of diguanides in obese non-diabetic women. *Lancet* ii, 13–15.

Nakra, B. R. S., Rutland, P., Verma, S. and Gaind, R. (1977). Amitriptyline and weight gain; a biochemical and endocrinological study. *Curr. Med. Res. Opin.* **4**, 602–608.

Noble, R. E. (1969). Effect of cyproheptadine on appetite and weight gain in adults. *J. Amer. Med. Ass.* **209**, 2054–2055.

Oswald, Z., Jones, H. S. and Mannerheim, J. E. (1968). Effects of two slimming drugs on sleep. *Brit. Med. J.* i, 796–799.

Oswald, Z., Lewis, S. A., Dunleavy, D. L. F., Brezinova, V. and Briggs, M. (1971). Drugs of dependence though not of abuse: fenfluramine and imipramine. *Brit. Med. J.* iii, 70–73.

Pawlowski, G. J. (1975). Cyproheptadine weight gain and appetite stimulation in essential anorexic adults. *Curr. Ther. Res.* **18**, 673–8.

Paykel, E. S., Muller, P. S. and de la Vergne, P. M. (1973). Amitriptyline, weight gain and carbohydrate craving: a side effect. *Br. J. Psychiat.* **123**, 501–507.

Penick, S. B. and Hinkle, L. (1963). The effect of glucagon, phenmetrazine and epineprine on hunger, food intake and plasma NEFA. *Amer. J. Clin. Nutr.* **13**, 110–114.

Penick, S. B. and Hinkle, L. E. (1964). Effect of expectation on response to phenmetrazine. *Psychosom. Med.* **26**, 369–373.

Penick, S. B., Smith, G. P., Wieneke, K. and Hinkle, L. E. (1963). Experimental evaluation between hunger and gastric motility. *Amer. J. Physiol.* **205**, 421–426.

Pinder, R. M., Brogden, R. N., Sawyer, P. R., Speight, T. M. and Avery, G. S. (1975). Fenfluramine: a review of its pharmacological properties and therapeutic efficacy in obesity and diabetes mellitus. *Drugs* **10** 241–323.

Printzmetal, M. and Alles, G. A. (1940). The central nervous system stimulant effects of dextroamphetamine sulphate. *Amer. J. Med. Sci.* **200**, 665–673.

Printzmetal, M. and Bloomberg, W. (1935). The use of benzedrine for the treatment of narcolepsy. *J. Amer. Med. Ass.* **105**, 2051–2054.

Pudel, V. E. (1976). Experimental feeding in man. *In* "Appetite and Food Intake" (T. Silverstone, ed.), pp. 245–264, Abakon, Berlin.

Quaade, F. and Jahl, O. (1962). Arterio-venous glucose and oxygen differences in cerebral blood of normal persons during hunger and satiety. *Amer. J. Med. Sci.* **243**, 438–445.

Robinson, R. G., McHugh, P. R. and Folstein, M. F. (1978). Measurement of appetite disturbance in psychiatric disorders. *J. Psychiat. Res.* **12**, 59–68.

Roginsky, M. S. and Barnett, J. (1966). Double-blind study of phenothyldiguanide (phenformin) on weight control of obese non-diabetic subjects. *Amer. J. Clin. Nut.* **19**, 223–226.

Saleh, J. W., Young, M. U., Van Italie, T. B. and Hashim, S. (1979). Ingestion behaviour and composition of weight change during cyproheptadine administration. *Int. J. Obesity* **3**, 213–222.

Schou, M., Baastrup, P., Grof, P., Weis, P. and Angst, J. (1970). Pharmacological and clinical problems of lithium prophylaxis. *Brit. J. Psychiat.* **116**, 615–619.

Seaton, D. A., Rose, K. and Duncan, L. J. P. (1964). A comparison of the appetite suppressing properties of d-amphetamine and phentermine. *Scot. Med. J.* **9**, 482–485.

Shoulson, Z. and Chase, T. N. (1975). Fenfluramine in man: hypophagia associated with diminished serotonin turnover. *Clin. Pharmacol. Ther.* **17**, 616–621.

Silverstone, J. T. (1968). The evaluation of appetite suppressant drugs. Paper presented at 3rd International Conference on the Regulation of Food and Water Intake, Philadelphia.

Silverstone, J. T. (1972). The anorectic effect of a long-acting preparation of phentermine (Duromine). *Psychopharmacologia* **25**, 315–320.

Silverstone, J. T. (1975). Anorectic drugs. *In* "Obesity: Pathogenesis and Management" (T. Silverstone, ed.), pp. 198–199, MTP, Lancaster.

Silverstone, J. T. and Besser, G. M. (1971). Insulin, blood sugar and hunger. *Postgrad. Med. J.* (June Suppl.), 427–429.

Silverstone, J. T. and Cleary, T. (1967). The treatment of obesity: a controlled trial of an evening dose of diethylpropion. *Clin. Trials. J.* (London), **4**, 837–840.

Silverstone, J. T., Fincham, J. and Campbell, D. B. (1975). The anorectic activity of fenfluramine. *Postgrad. Med. J.* **51**, Suppl. 1, 171–174.

Silverstone, J. T., Fincham, J. and Plumley, J. (1979). An evaluation of the anorectic activity in man of a sustained release formulation of tiflorex. *Brit. J. Clin. Pharmacol.* **7**, 353–356.

Silverstone, J. T., Fincham, J., Wells, B. and Kyriakides, M. (1980). The effect of pimozide on amphetamine induced arousal, euphoria and anorexia in man. *Neuropharmacology*.

Silverstone, J. T. and Schuyler, D. (1975). The effect of cyproheptadine on hunger, calorie intake and body weight in man. *Psychopharmacologia* **40**, 335–340.

Silverstone, J. T. and Stunkard, A. J. (1968). The anorectic effect of dexamphetamine sulphate. *Brit. J. Pharmacol. Chemother.* **33**, 513–522.

Silverstone, J. T., Turner, P. and Humpherson, P. L. (1968). Direct measurement of the anorectic activity of diethylpropion. *J. Clin. Pharmacol.* **8**, 172–179.

Silverstone, J. T. and Wells, B. (1980). Clinical psychopharmacology of amphetamine and related compounds. *In* "Amphetamine and Related Stimulants" (J. Caldwell, ed.), CRC Press, Boca Raton, Florida.

Simeons, A. J. W. (1954). The action of chorionic gonadotrophin in the obese. *Lancet* **i**, 946–947.

Sjoberg, L. and Jonsson, C. O. (1967). Studies in the psychological effects of a new drug (diethylpropion). *Scan. J. Psychol.* **8**, 81–87.

Smart, J. V. and Turner, P. (1966). Influence of urinary pH on the degree and duration of action of amphetamine on the critical flicker fusion frequency in man. *Brit. J. Pharmacol. Chemother.* **26**, 468–472.

Smart, J. V., Sneddon, J. M. and Turner, P. (1967). A comparison of the effects of chlorphentermine, diethylpropion and phentermine on critical flicker frequency. *Brit. J. Pharmacol. Chemother.* **30**, 307–316.

Smith, G. M. and Beecher, H. K. (1959). Amphetamine sulphate and athletic performance. 1. Objective effects. *J. Amer. Med. Ass.* **170**, 524–557.

Smith, G. M. and Beecher, H. K. (1964). Drugs and judgement: effects of amphetamine and secobarbital on self-stimulation. *J. Psychol.* **58**, 397–405.

Smith, G. M., Weitzner, M., Levenson, S. R. and Beecher, H. K. (1963). Effects of amphetamine and secobarbital on coding and mathematical performance. *J. Pharmacol.* **141**, 100–104.

Smith, R. C. and Davis, J. M. (1977). Comparative effects of d-amphetamine, l-amphetamine and methylphendiate on mood in man. *Psychopharmacology* **53**, 1–12.

Smith, R. G., Innes, J. A. and Munro, J. F. (1975). Double-blind evaluation of mazindol in refractory obesity. *Brit. Med. J.* iii, 284.

Stacher, G., Bauer, H. and Steminger, H. (1979). Cholesystokinin decreases appetite and activation evoked by stimuli arising from preparation of a meal in man. *Physiol. Behav.* 23, 325–332.

Sturdevant, R. A. L. and Goetz, H. (1976). Cholesystokinin both stimulates and inhibits human food intake. *Nature* 261, 713–715.

Turner, P. (1971). Further studies on the human pharmacology of fenfluramine. *S. Afr. Med. J.* 45, Suppl, 13, 13.

Turner, P. (1978). How do anti-obesity drugs work? *Int. J. Obesity* 2, 343–348.

Turner, P. (1979). Peripheral mechanisms of action of fenfluramine. *Curr. Med. Res. Opin.* 6, Suppl. 1, 101–106.

Valiente, S., Bahamondes, G. and Toro, A. (1967). Effect of cyproheptadine on body weight. *Bol. Hosp. S. Juan.* (Santiago) 14, 342–346.

Vendsborg, P. B. and Rafaelson, O. J. (1973). Lithium in man: effect on glucose tolerance and serum electrolytes. *Acta. Psychiat. Scan.* 49, 601–610.

Weiss, B. and Laties, V. G. (1962). Enhancement of human performance by caffeine and the amphetamines. *Pharmacol. Reviews* 14, 1–35.

Wooley, O. R., Wooley, S. L. and Lee, J. C. (1979). The effect of fenfluramine on appetite for palatable food in humans. *Curr. Med. Res. Opin.* 6, Suppl. 1, 83–90.

# 6 □ Drug Treatment of Obesity

J. F. Munro and M. J. Ford

## INTRODUCTION

Although many ascribe the development of obesity to either gluttony or sloth, the evidence that the obese take less exercise or eat more than the non-obese remains anecdotal. Indeed, the converse might be true (Garrow, 1978). It seems probable that the aetiology of obesity is complex and multifactorial. However, the adipose tissue mass can only be reduced when energy expenditure exceeds intake. This can be achieved either by increasing expenditure or by reducing intake. As the energy value of 1 kg of adipose tissue is about 7000 kcal (29.4 MJ), an energy gap of 500 kcals (2.1 MJ) should promote a weight loss of 0.5 kg/week or 26 kg in the year. In practice, such a loss is unlikely to be maintained because weight reduction itself will lead to a fall in energy expenditure and may thus close the energy gap (James et al., 1979).

The currently available anti-obesity drugs either act peripherally by increasing energy expenditure (such as thyroxine) or in some other manner (such as the biguanides), or are primarily "appetite suppressants", and act by exerting a central effect on appetite or satiety.

In a survey of 1000 slimmers conducted by the Consumer's Association, half had seen their general practitioner with their weight problem and of these, half had been given an appetite reducing drug (Which ? Way to Slim, 1978). Current estimates suggest that although the number of prescriptions has recently fallen in the UK, it remains at about 2½ million per annum. This figure would imply either these drugs have an important role to play in the management of obesity, or that they are being extensively overprescribed. The ideal anti-obesity agent should be effective, devoid of adverse effects, including the potential for drug dependence, and have additional beneficial effects on obesity-related diseases. Not surprisingly, no such agent exists. At present, anti-obesity drug therapy remains a compromise between the efficacy and side-effects of drug therapy on the one hand, and the need to promote or maintain weight reduction on the other. The point at which this compromise is reached for a given patient is unique to that individual.

The appetite suppressant preparations which are available on prescription in the UK are shown in Table I with details of the recommended daily dosage (MIMS 1980). All but mazindol are structurally related to amphetamine (Fig. 1). Their central mode of action has been extensively discussed in previous chapters. This chapter describes their clinical application and attempts to answer the following questions:

(1) Can anti-obesity drugs be given with reasonable safety?
(2) Do they promote weight loss and/or prevent weight regain?
(3) What happens when therapy is discontinued?
(4) Can prolonged treatment ever be justified?

*Table I.* Antiobesity drugs currently available in the UK.

| Formulation | Proprietary names | Recommended dosage (mg/day) |
|---|---|---|
| [a]Amphetamine Resin Complex | Durophet | 12.5 mg |
| [a]Phenmetrazine (30 mg) Phenbutrazate (20 mg) | Filon | 2 tablets |
| Phentermine | Duromine Ionamin | 30 mg |
| Diethylpropion | Tenuate Apisate | 75 mg |
| Mazindol | Teronac | 2 mg |
| Fenfluramine | Ponderax | 120 mg |

[a]  Restricted use under Schedule 2 of the "Misuse of Drugs" Act 1971 (Mims, 1980).

## PHARMACOKINETICS AND SIDE-EFFECTS

### Amphetamine

Amphetamine is a racemic compound comprising equal portions of the dextro- and laevo-isomers. Both are completely absorbed within 2–3 h of oral administration, have a plasma half-life of about 5 h and are excreted in the urine substantially unchanged at a rate closely dependent upon the urinary pH (Morselli *et al.*, 1978; Beckett, 1979). As sympathomimetic amines, the central stimulating effects are marked, the dextro-isomer being four times more potent than the laevo-isomer and twice as potent as the racemic compound (Printzmetal and Alles, 1940). In the short term, these effects result in increased alertness, lowered fatigue, elevation of mood and appetite suppression. However, the euphoriant property of the amphetamines has led to their widespread abuse and high dependence liability in vulnerable personalities (Isbell and Chrusciel, 1970; Csillag, 1971).

Common side-effects include insomnia, restlessness, irritability, tremor, excess perspiration, dry mouth, epigastric discomfort, constipation and palpitations. Though transient elevations in blood pressure may occur following acute administration, in the longer term, no significant alteration in blood pressure is observed though this may reflect the opposing effect of weight loss. Chronic amphetamine abuse may result in anxiety and confusional states, paranoid psychoses and even permanent brain damage (Connell, 1975). Deaths have also been reported from acidental and deliberate self-poisoning.

## Phenmetrazine

Phenmetrazine is well absorbed, rapidly metabolized and excreted by the biliary and renal tracts. Its anorectic and euphoriant properties are similar to those of amphetamine though it has less central and cardiac-stimulating effects (Spillane, 1960; Fletcher et al., 1961). Its adverse effects are also similar, namely insomnia, restlessness, irritability, tremor, tachycardia, dry mouth and epigastric discomfort. Acute or chronic confusional and psychotic states have been reported (Evans, 1959; Connell, 1975), and it is contra-indicated in anxiety states and thyrotoxicosis.

## Phentermine

Phentermine is a weak sympathomimetic drug which is well absorbed from the small intestine, has a plasma half-life of 20–24 h and is excreted in the urine both unchanged and as inactive metabolites. The rate of absorption is considerably slower for the resinate compound than for soluble salts and the urinary excretion is pH-dependent (Hinsvack, 1973).

Given as a sustained release resin complex, therapeutic levels are obtained within 1 h of oral administration and persist for at least 20 h. Animal studies have shown inotropic, chronotropic and vasopressor cardiac effects (Yelnosky et al., 1969). In man however, possibly because of the coincidental weight loss associated with its clinical use, no significant changes in blood pressure have been recorded though transient increases in blood pressure may occur following acute administration (Morselli et al., 1978; Le Riche, 1960).

Adverse drug effects do occur, but only rarely require withdrawal of the drug; they include insomnia, nervousness, nausea, dry mouth and constipation.

## Diethylpropion

The amphetamine congener, diethylpropion, is well absorbed producing peak levels within 2 h of oral administration. It exhibits first pass kinetics with rapid hepatic metabolism to active metabolites. It is these and not the parent drug which are responsible for the pharmacological effects. Diethylpropion is therefore twice as potent when administered orally than parenterally (Jasinski et al., 1974; Wright et al., 1975). The elimination half-life of its active metabolites is about 8 h.

In animals, the cardiac and vasopressor effects of diethylpropion are less than those of amphetamine. Indeed, it has been given intravenously to patients with hypertension or ischaemic heart disease without producing adverse cardiac effects (Alfaro *et al.*, 1960). The central stimulant properties in man are only 10–20% of those of amphetamine (Hoekenga *et al.*, 1978). The adverse drug effects are usually mild but include insomnia, restlessness, dry mouth, constipation. Psychotic illnesses have been reported on rare occasions following its administration (*Med. J. Aust.*, 1970).

## Mazindol

In spite of the chemical dissimilarity, mazindol behaves pharmacologically as an amphetamine congener. It has cardiac and vasopressor effects and produces central stimulation (Gogerty *et al.*, 1968; Hadler, 1972; Bradley, 1974). The pharmacokinetics in man are difficult to evaluate since the drug and its metabolites cannot be readily distinguished. Peak drug levels occur 2 h after administration and coincide with the onset of the anorectic effect. The elimination half-life is about 50 h though the true half-lives of the active drug or metabolites are unknown (Sandoz Pharmaceuticals, 1973).

Because it may potentiate the pressor effects of catecholamines, it should never be used in conjunction with sympathomimetic drugs or adrenergic neuron-blocking antihypertensive compounds such as debrisoquine and bethanidine. It is contra-indicated in hyperthyroidism, anxiety states and peptic ulceration. Adverse effects are not infrequent and include insomnia, nervousness, dizziness, dry mouth, nausea and constipation. Angioneurotic oedema, vomiting with peripheral oedema and violent tremors in a patient taking methyldopa and flurazepam have also been reported (Wallace, 1976; Maclay and Wallace, 1977).

## Fenfluramine

Fenfluramine is rapidly absorbed with an absorption half-life of approximately 1 h. It has a plasma half-life of about 20 h and after multiple dosage, steady state levels are achieved within four to five days. Both fenfluramine and its active metabolite, norfenfluramine, are excreted by the renal tract with an elimination rate which is pH-dependent (Campbell, 1971). Though animal studies have shown a vasopressor effect, particularly on the pulmonary circulation, as in the use of amphetamines, the weight loss produced is frequently associated with a fall in blood pressure (Yelnosky and Lawlor, 1970; Follows, 1971). Furthermore, it has been suggested that fenfluramine has a mild hypotensive effect independent of weight loss and will enhance the effect of concomitation antihypertensive drug therapy (Waal-Manning and Simpson, 1969; Boledeoku *et al.*, 1972). Fenfluramine exerts depressant rather than stimulant central effects differing markedly in this respect from the amphetamines (Fink *et al.*, 1971).

Adverse drug effects are common. They include dry mouth, drowsiness, lethargy, light-headedness and diarrhoea. Less commonly, fenfluramine may produce nausea, irritability, depression and depersonalization. Like amphetamine, it suppresses REM sleep and may reduce the quality and duration of sleep, causing insomnia with nightmares (Gagnon *et al.*, 1969). Fenfluramine withdrawal may produce depression in susceptible individuals and for this reason, it should always be reduced gradually over several days before therapy is stopped. Like other phenylethylamines, fenfluramine should not be administered to patients with a history of glaucoma, epilepsy or depression. It should also be avoided in patients who are taking or have recently stopped taking monoamineoxidase inhibitors.

## SAFETY

Analysis of ten commonly reported side-effects of the anti-obesity drugs reveals a high frequency of complaints of insomnia, nervousness and dry mouth with amphetamine, phenmetrazine and phentermine, and of lethargy, dizziness and diarrhoea with fenfluramine (Table II). In addition, interrogation of patients previously treated with an anorectic agent revealed that almost half those receiving amphetamine reported unpleasant side-effects, as did 44% of those taking mazindol and 42% of subjects treated with phenmetrazine. The reported incidences with phentermine, fenfluramine and diethylpropion were 31%, 30% and 27% respectively (Ashwell, 1973). In addition, the Dawn Reports 1973–75 and 1976, emphasized the potential for drug abuse with amphetamine and to a lesser extent, phenmetrazine, especially among teenagers (Carabillo, 1978) (Tables III and IV). Both these drugs are now controlled in the UK by the Misuse of Drugs Act 1971 and by comparable regulations in some other countries. Although drug abuse is rarely found in the obese patient, we believe that the general risk of abuse by others is such that their continued availability as anorectic agents for the treatment of obesity is not justified.

Because of their euphoriant effects, there is also a potential for drug abuse with phentermine and diethylpropion; indeed, the latter may have been manufactured illegally for sale as a stimulant drug. However, abuse is rare and probably restricted to those already addicted to other drugs (Cohen, 1977; Carabillo, 1978). The only reports of fenfluramine abuse have occurred in established drug addicts (Levin, 1975), and its non-stimulant properties are such that the potential for abuse must be extremely low. The recognized hazards of mazindol, fenfluramine, phentermine and diethylpropion may restrict their use to selected patients but in such patients, their administration may be justified provided they can be shown to be effective.

## CLINICAL EFFICACY

There is considerable evidence that the "appetite suppressant" drugs will promote weight loss. From an analysis of 160 double-blind studies involving 7725 patients, the Food & Drug Administration Working Party reported that

*Table II.* Percentage incidence of adverse drug effects on the recommended dosage of antiobesity drugs.

| Adverse effect | Amphetamine | Phenmetrazine | Phentermine | Diethylpropion | Mazindol | Fenfluramine | Placebo |
|---|---|---|---|---|---|---|---|
| Source | Seaton et al., 1964; Vernace 1974. | Poindexter, 1960; Shapiro and Bogran, 1960. | Steel et al., 1973; Seaton et al., 1964; Truant et al., 1972. | Noble, 1971; G.P. research group, 1978. | G.P. research group 1978; Vernace 1974; Asher W. L. (Personal communication) | Pinder et al., 1975. | Steel et al., |
| Insomnia | 12 | 12 | 6 | 6 | 6 | 2 | 2 |
| Nervousness | 8 | 20 | 14 | 4 | 3 | 6 | 4 |
| Lethargy | 3 | 4 | 8 | 2 | 4 | 15 | 3 |
| Depression | 1 | 1 | 1 | — | — | 3 | 1 |
| Dizziness | 6 | 6 | 9 | 1 | 3 | 10 | 1 |
| Dry Mouth | 22 | 10 | 17 | 5 | 7 | 6 | 3 |
| Nausea | 8 | 5 | 4 | 4 | 7 | 6 | 1 |
| Constipation | 8 | 6 | 8 | 6 | 3 | — | 4 |
| Diarrhoea | — | — | — | — | — | 13 | 2 |
| Palpitations (Rapid Pulse) | 2 | 3 | — | 3 | 2 | — | 1 |

(Adapted from Bray and Greenway 1976.)

*Table III.* Misuse of the Antiobesity Drugs
(Dawn Reports 1973–1975).

| Drug | Reports per million prescriptions |
|------|-----------------------------------|
| Amphetamine | 45.3 |
| Phenmetrazine | 5.7 |
| Phentermine | 1.7 |
| Diethylpropion | 1.3 |
| Mazindol | 0.7 |
| Fenfluramine | 1.6 |

(Adapted from Carabillo 1978.)

*Table IV.* Misuse of the antiobesity drugs.

| | | | Motives for misuse | | |
|---|---|---|---|---|---|
| [a] Dawn Reports (1976) | Antiobesity drug market | Antiobesity drug misuse problem | Stimulant effect | Dependence state | Others or unknown |
| Phenmetrazine | 13% | 50% | 31% | 53% | 16% |
| Diethylpropion | 44% | 31% | 75% | 1% | 24% |
| Phentermine | 24% | 12% | 55% | 4% | 41% |
| Mazindol | 10% | 1% | 47% | 7% | 46% |
| Fenfluramine | 9% | 6% | 67% | 2% | 31% |

[a] Excluding all other anorectic drugs (Adapted from Carabillo, 1978).

in over 90% of the studies, drugs produced greater weight loss than placebo, though in only 40% of the studies was the difference statistically significant. The overall weight loss attributable to drug therapy was 0.2 kg (0.5 lb) per week (Scoville, 1973). In the long term, this might imply a substantial benefit.

However, the majority of studies analysed were for a limited duration and even so, the default rates were high, accounting for almost half the patients. The rate of mean weight loss varied considerably between studies, but the Working Party considered the major variables related to factors other than the drug used, such as patient selection and the dietary advice given. This is not surprising as patients seeking medical help for a weight problem comprise a very mixed group. Some may wish to reduce for cosmetic reasons, others may have a pressing medical need. Some will be trying to reduce for the first time, while others will have tried numerous previous therapies. In an attempt to minimize these differences in patient selection, an Edinburgh group have studied female patients with "Refractory Obesity" as defined by the following criteria:

(1)  Excess weight in the absence of oedema of at least 20%.

(2)  Previous regular attendance at a hospital obesity clinic for at least 12 months.

(3)  Previous dietary advice given to provide a daily calorie intake of 1000 k cal (4.2 MJ) based on the principle of carbohydrate restriction.

(4)  Failure to lose weight during the 3 months prior to the study.

(5)  No anti-obesity drug therapy for at least 3 months prior to the study.

The results of anorectic drug therapy in comparable groups of patients with refractory obesity are shown in Table V. In these studies, the overall attrition rate attributable to therapy was reduced to 9% on placebo and 10% on active treatment. During the first 4 weeks of each study, the mean weight change attributable to drug therapy was comparable to that reported by the F.D.A. However, with the possible exception of fenfluramine, the rate of mean weight loss was markedly reduced by week 8, producing a new mean plateau weight.

The conclusions of the F.D.A. Working Party and the studies in refractory obesity provide indirect evidence of the comparability of the weight-reducing properties of the available drugs. Further evidence is provided from double-blind comparative studies of at least 12 weeks duration in patients also given dietary instruction. The results of six such studies are summarized in Table VI.

Although the mean rate of weight loss varied from one study to another, the differences in weight loss achieved by the drugs undergoing comparison was only once greater than 0.1 kg/week, and that particular trial, a comparison of diethylpropion with mazindol, can however be criticized on the grounds that in spite of its title, it was not double-blind in design! (General Practitioner Research Group, 1978).

Generally speaking, the evidence would suggest that the available drugs are roughly equal in efficacy and the choice of drug should be influenced by such factors as the nature and frequency of side-effects and cost.


## MODE OF ADMINISTRATION

Because of the possible development of drug tolerance and the risk of drug abuse, a number of double-blind studies have compared continuous and intermittent therapy with amphetamine, diethylpropion, mazindol and fenfluramine over periods ranging from 12 to 36 weeks (Table VII).

In many instances, intermittent therapy comprised 4 weeks of drug treatment alternating with 4 weeks of placebo therapy. There is however, no special reason to suggest that this is an optimum regime. Intermittent fenfluramine was less effective than continuous treatment and was associated with a much higher incidence of adverse side-effects, especially withdrawal depression (Steel and Briggs, 1972). For this reason, it cannot be recommended. Using the other drugs, the benefit of continuous therapy on weight loss is only marginal and we would recommend intermittent treatment since it is less costly and presumably less likely to be associated with drug dependence or abuse.

Table V. Double-blind studies in refractory obesity.

| Data | Pooled placebo | Amphetamine | Phentermine | Diethylpropion | Mazindol | Fenfluramine |
|---|---|---|---|---|---|---|
| Source | a | Seaton et al., 1964 | Seaton et al., 1964 | Seaton et al., 1961 | Smith et al., 1975 | Munro et al., 1966 |
| Duration | 12 | 12 | 12 | 12 | 12 | 12 |
| Dosage (mg/day) | — | 15 | 30 | 100 | 2 | 80 |
| Number completing study | 140 | 21 | 21 | 40 | 19 | 20 |
| Number of drop-outs | 12 | 4 | 0 | 4 | 6 | 5 |
| Mean age (years) | 52 | 58 | 57 | 54 | 47 | 49 |
| Mean % excess weight | 46 | 41 | 43 | 42 | 53 | 45 |
| Maximum individual weight loss (kg) | 5.9 | 6.8 | 6.8 | 4.5 | 8.6 | 9.1 |
| Mean rate of weight loss (kg/wk) | 0 | 0.2 | 0.2 | 0.1 | 0.1 | 0.3 |
| Cumulative mean weight losses (kg) | | | | | | |
| week 4 | 0.3 | 1.5 | 2.0 | 1.2 | 1.7 | 2.0 |
| week 8 | +0.2 | 2.7 | 2.5 | 1.4 | 1.3 | 3.4 |
| Week 12 | +0.3 | 2.9 | 2.7 | 1.2 | 1.4 | 4.2 |

aNo placebo group used in the comparative study of amphetamine and phentermine.

*Table VI.* Double-blind comparative studies in obesity.

| Drugs | Dosage (mg/day) | Source | Dietary regimen | Duration (wks) | Number completing study | Mean rate of weight loss (kg/week) |
|---|---|---|---|---|---|---|
| Amphetamine | 15 | Seaton et al., 1964 | Simple restriction | 12 | 42 | 0.2 |
| Phentermine | 30 | | | | | 0.2 |
| Amphetamine | 15 | Vernace, 1974 | 1000 cal. | 12 | 64 | 0.5 |
| Mazindol | 3 | | | | | 0.5 |
| Phentermine[a] | 30 | Steel et al., 1973 | 1000 cal. | 36 | 63 | 0.3 |
| Fenfluramine | 60 | | | | | 0.3 |
| Diethylpropion | 75 | G.P. research group, 1978 | Simple restriction | 16 | 76 | 0.4 |
| Mazindol | 2 | | | | | 0.6 |
| Diethylpropion | 75 | Hoekenga et al., 1978 | Simple restriction | 12 | 31 | 0.4 |
| Fenfluramine | 60 | | | | | 0.5 |
| Mazindol | 2 | Gomez, 1975 | Simple restriction | 12 | 58 | 0.5 |
| Fenfluramine | 60 | | | | | 0.4 |

[a] Used intermittently during alternate 4-week periods.

Although the studies with refractory obesity have shown that the mean weight loss plateaus within a few weeks of initiating treatment, it can be argued that the additional weight loss attributable to drug treatment might be increased if this was initiated before the development of refractory obesity. This suggestion can be tested by analysing the results of double-blind studies of similar duration administered to unselected subjects (Table VII). Such an analysis reveals an overall mean weight loss attributable to drug therapy ranging from 0.2 kg to 0.5 kg/week. However, during the last 4 weeks of therapy, the additional benefit of drug treatment is much reduced implying that a plateauing effect has again occurred within a few weeks of starting treatment.

Indeed, a recent extensive review of the outpatient management of obesity found that drug therapy failed to produce weight losses in excess of those achieved by other means and that behavioural therapy was best at maintaining weight loss (Wing and Jeffrey, 1979). It is possible that the results can be improved by combining drug treatment with group therapy (London and Schreiber, 1966). A few studies have evaluated the possibility of combining drug treatment with behavioural modification. One has shown that the combination of phentermine with behavioural therapy produced greater weight losses than that achieved by the drug or behavioural therapy alone (Brightwell and Naylor, 1979). Similar results have been reported using fenfluramine though weight regain occurred when the drug was discontinued, whether or not it had been given in combination with behavioural therapy (Stunkard and Brownell, 1979). It has been sugggested that the behavioural modification programme should be so structured as to make optimum use of the pharmacological effects of the drug. Thus while using fenfluramine, the subject should be instructed to eat small meals slowly (Blundell et al., 1979). Combined therapy justifies further evaluation.

## SELECTION OF PATIENTS

These various studies might suggest that the benefits for anorectic drug therapy are insubstantial and outweighed by the hazards of treatment. However so far, we have only considered mean weight losses. Within every study, there is a very considerable variety in individual response. Although in part this will reflect patient selection, even among subjects with refractory obesity, there is a wide range of weight change, with maximal weight losses ranging from 0.4 kg/week on diethylpropion to 0.6 kg/week on fenfluramine (see Table V).

One obvious factor that will influence the result of any drug treatment is patient compliance. In some instances, failure to reduce might merely reflect poor compliance possibly attributable to drug-induced side-effects. The variability in patient response, however, might also reflect fundamental differences in drug metabolism and pharmacokinetics. In order to test this possi-

Silverstone 56

*Table VII.* Continuous *vs* intermittent therapy in unselected obese subjects on 1000 calorie diet.

| Drug | Dosage (mg/day) | Source | Intermittent regimen active: placebo (weeks) | Duration | Number completing study | Mean rate of weight loss (kg/week) | | |
|---|---|---|---|---|---|---|---|---|
| | | | | | | Placebo | Inter-mittent | Continuous |
| Amphetamine | 12.5 | Silverstone and Lascelles, 1965 | 4:4 | 16 | 32 | 0.3 | 0.4 | 0.6 |
| Phentermine | 30 | Truant *et al.*, 1972 | 3:1 | 16 | 56 | 0.3 | 0.5 | 0.6 |
| | 30 | Munro *et al.*, 1968 | 4:4 | 36 | 64 | 0.1 | 0.4 | 0.3 |
| Diethylpropion | 75 | Nolan, 1975 | 4:4 | 12 | 51 | 0.4 | 0.5 | 0.6 |
| | 75 | McQuarrie, 1975 | 4:4 | 12 | 61 | 0.1 | 0.3 | 0.4 |
| | 75 | Allen, 1975 | 4:4 | 12 | 86 | 0.4 | 0.6 | 0.8 |
| | 75 | Silverstone, 1974 | 4:4 | 16 | 81 | — | 0.4 | 0.5 |
| | 75 | Le Riche and Cisma, 1967 | 4:4 | 24 | 36 | — | 0.5 | 0.3 |
| Mazindol | 3 | Conte, 1973 | 4:2 | 16 | 69 | 0.2 | 0.3 | 0.4 |
| | 3 | Asher W.L. (personal communication) | 4:2 | 16 | 79 | 0.2 | 0.5 | 0.4 |
| Fenfluramine | 60 | Steel *et al.*, 1973 | 4:4 | 36 | 50 | — | 0.2 | 0.3 |

Table VIII. Double-blind studies in unselected obese subjects on 1000 calorie diet.

| Data | Amphetamine | Phentermine | Diethylpropion | Mazindol | Fenfluramine |
|---|---|---|---|---|---|
| Source | Vernace 1974 | Langlois et al., 1974 | McQuarrie, 1975 | Maclay and Wallace, 1977 | Hudson, 1977 |
| Duration (wks) | 12 | 14 | 12 | 12 | 12 |
| Dosage (mg/day) | 15 | 30 | 75 | 2 | 80 |
| Nos completing study | | | | | |
| active | 32 | 30 | 22 | 155 | 176 |
| placebo | 33 | 29 | 19 | 137 | 15 |
| Mean weight loss (kg) | | | | | |
| active | 5.9 | 7.3 | 4.4 | 7.2 | 7.6 |
| placebo | 2.6 | 1.8 | 1.5 | 4.6 | 5.6 |
| Mean additional rate of weight loss (kg/week) | | | | | |
| weeks 1–4 | 0.3 | 0.5 | 0.2 | 0.2 | 0.2 |
| weeks 4–8 | 0.4 | 0.6 | 0.5 | 0.4 | 0.2 |
| weeks 8–12 | 0.2 | 0.1 | 0.1 | 0.1 | 0.0 |

bility, a group of patients with refractory obesity were given fenfluramine for 20 weeks increasing the dose gradually up to a maximum of 160 mg/day or until the development of troublesome side-effects. Once a stable dosage regime had been achieved, plasma fenfluramine and norfenfluramine concentrations were measured, and for each subject, the mean drug concentration was estimated. Analysis of the data confirmed that there was a significant relationship between weight loss and plasma drug concentration (Innes *et al.*, 1977) (see Table IX).

*Table IX.* Rate of weight loss and plasma fenfluramine concentration.

|  | Plasma Fenfluramine (ng/ml) | | |
| --- | --- | --- | --- |
| Data (Innes *et al.*, 1977) | 0–99 | 100–199 | 200–299 |
| Number completing 20 weeks | 13 | 15 | 13 |
| Mean % excess weight | 59 | 54 | 51 |
| Mean dosage (mg/day) | 124 | 130 | 148 |
| Mean plasma fenfluramine (ng/ml) | 78 | 148 | 239 |
| Mean rate of weight loss (kg/week) | 0.11 | 0.25 | 0.44 |
| Weeks 0–8 | 0.3 | 0.4 | 0.6 |
| Weeks 8–12 | 0.1 | 0.3 | 0.7 |
| Weeks 12–16 | 0.1 | 0.1 | 0.3 |

Moreover, a satisfactory mean rate of weight loss was maintained throughout the study period by those subjects whose plasma concentrations were in excess of 200 $\mu$g/ml. It remains to be seen whether or not comparable results can be obtained with other agents. However, subsequent experience has shown that some subjects will fail to lose weight even with plasma fenfluramine concentrations considerably greater than 200 $\mu$g/ml. It follows that although variables in drug absorption, distribution or metabolism may be important in explaining the unpredictability of drug therapy, they are not the only factors.

This is not surprising. Unpredictability of response is not restricted to drug therapy. Some might argue that the individual response to any form of treatment is influenced by the controversial question of whether the subject has "hypertrophic" or "hyperplastic" obesity, because it has been suggested that the former is more resistant to weight reduction (Krotkiewski *et al.*, 1977). It seems probable that the uncertainty of individual response to treatment will only be clarified by a greater understanding of the aetiology of obesity, and the metabolic consequences of weight change (Danforth *et al.*, 1978). In the meantime, however, we can arbitrarily divide obese subjects into four categories:

(1) Those with a "normal" energy expenditure who can curtail their intake sufficiently to create an effective energy gap without recourse to drug therapy.

(2) Those with a "normal" energy expenditure who find it impossible to curb their food consumption without the addition of a drug influencing appetite or satiety.

(3) Those with a "normal" energy expenditure who find it impossible to curb their food consumption even when given an 'appetite suppressant".

(4) Those in whom the basic problem is one of energy expenditure, so much so, that in spite of controlling intake, they are unable to achieve effective weight loss.

Clearly, the centrally acting drugs are unneccesary in the first category, ineffective in the third and also likely to be largely ineffective in the fourth. Their use should therefore be restricted to the second category, but at present, there is no means of identifying these patients other than by assessing their response to drug treatment.

## DURATION OF TREATMENT AND EFFECTS OF DRUG WITHDRAWAL

In a survey of 450 American doctors, 88% of the general practitioners questioned, and 50% of the hospital internists prescribed appetite suppressants. Of these however, only 25% prescribed such drugs for longer than 12 weeks (Lasagna, 1973). Clinical experience would suggest that most obese subjects rapidly regain weight as soon as drug therapy is discontinued and that the degree of weight regained roughly parallels the loss achieved during treatment. This is supported by the evidence from short-term cross-over studies when subjects received placebo therapy following active treatment (Lawson *et al.*, 1970; Carney and Tweddell, 1975; Haugen, 1975; Miach *et al.*, 1976; Brightwell and Naylor, 1979). Only a handful of studies have reported the more long-term consequences of stopping therapy (Langlois *et al.*, 1974; Vernace, 1974; Hudson, 1977; Gotestam, 1979). Again, the results support the contention that none of the currently available drugs produces a lasting effect on eating habit and that the weight loss that they induce is only temporary. It follows that their prescription for a conventional period of 12 weeks or so can only be justified in those patients who will achieve a greater than average degree of weight loss and even amongst these, only if there is a clearly defined short-term benefit. This could be psychological, e.g. prior to an important social function but more often, is physical, e.g. before an elective operation such as cholecystectomy.

## LONG-TERM THERAPY AND DRUG TOLERANCE

The evidence so far presented would imply that these drugs are currently being overprescribed or at least, inappropriately prescribed.

If weight regain following drug withdrawal is to be avoided, the price that may have to be paid is their long-term administration. The evidence that such an approach might prove effective is largely anecdotal (Smith, 1962; Craddock, 1973; Matthews, 1975). A number of studies have evalued drugs for 9 months or longer (Silverstone and Solomon, 1965; Munro et al., 1968; Steel et al., 1973; Enzi et al., 1976; Hudson, 1977). As expected, the mean weight losses are relatively disappointing; the rate of weight loss is maximal during the first 3 months and the only study in which substantial weight loss occurred after 6 months, is unusual because not only was there a loss of 4.9 kg on the active preparation (mazindol) but also of 3.0 kg on placebo therapy. The remarkable study of 176 patients by Hudson (1977) is of particular interest. Continuous fenfluramine administration produced a mean weight loss of 10.0 kg after 6 months, during the following 6 months, the further mean weight loss was only 0.4 kg. At this stage, the drug was discontinued, and during the following year, there was a mean weight regain of 8.9 kg. This study alone does not resolve the problem, but certainly it suggests that weight regain can be prevented by continuous drug therapy. This is contrary to the common practice of discontinuing the drug when weight loss ceases on the grounds that drug tolerance has developed.

While it would be foolhardy to suggest that true pharmacological tolerance may not occur—it is well-documented in animals (Opitz, 1978)—the fall-off in weight loss observed during anorectic drug treatment in obese patients may well be largely due to non-pharmacological factors (Silverstone, 1974). However, once true tolerance has developed, weight regain might be expected in spite of continuing treatment. Hudson has shown that this does not happen. Instead, it could be argued that the drug is continuing to exert an effect on food intake, but the energy gap necessary to promote weight loss has been closed because of the reduction in energy expenditure brought about by the combination of weight loss itself and of the metabolic adaptation to energy deprivation. The degree to which this adaptation can occur may in itself partly explain the variability in patient response not only to drug therapy but also to other therapeutic regimes. Indeed, it could even be compared with the plateauing effect in body weight that occurs about 2 years after a successful small bowel by-pass operation. Such a plateauing reflects the metabolic adaptation to energy deprivation, and rapid weight regain will occur if normal bowel continuity is restored.

However, it remains to be established whether or not life-long drug therapy will prove effective in preventing weight regain. Some might argue that the risks of this approach are unacceptable. Most would agree that such treatment could only be justified in those patients in whom the initial period of drug treatment had produced substantial weight loss in subjects who, for one reason or another, were at special risk because of their obesity. As the risk increases with the degree of obesity, long-term therapy could be most readily justified in the most overweight. This may be especially the case in men under the age of forty in whom uncomplicated obesity can be shown to influence life expectancy (Berchtold et al., 1977; Garrow, 1979). Others at special medical risk include the obese hypertensive and the obese diabetic whereas the combination of obesity with depression may create a vicious circle situation with compulsive eating causing further weight gain and aggravating the depression. The present and potential role of drug therapy in these high-risk situations is now considered.

## OBESITY AND DEPRESSION

Both obesity and depression are common conditions. They may not be causally related but they can certainly co-exist. Because of its side-effects, fenfluramine is probably contra-indicated and, with the possible exception of mazindol, the other appetite-suppressant drugs should also be avoided in the severely depressed. The antidepressant value of therapy with the tricyclic compounds such as amitriptyline, may be offset by the associated weight gain. A drug which combined anti-obesity and antidepressant properties would be particularly attractive as a long-term therapeutic agent. Two such preparations are currently undergoing evaluation.

### Ciclazindol

Ciclazindol is a tetracylic antidepressant which is structurally related to mazindol. *In vitro*, it increases glucose uptake in skeletal muscle (Kirby and Turner, 1977). As an antidepressant, it acts by inhibiting noradrenaline uptake and it is of comparable efficacy to amitriptyline (Ghose *et al.*, 1978). Its side-effects include tiredness, headaches and dizziness. Given to obese, non-depressed subjects, it produces a mean weight loss of 3.1 kg in 3 weeks (Greenbaum, 1979). In a comparative study, 60% of depressed patients taking ciclazindol lost weight compared with only 10% on amitriptyline (Levine, 1979).

### Zimelidine

Zimelidine is a bicyclic antidepressant which is a potent inhibitor of 5-hydroxytryptamine uptake. Unpublished clinical trials in non-depressed obese patients appear promising. It also has antidepressant properties comparable to amitriptyline though may be less likely to produce adverse side-effects. In a 4-week double-blind study in obese depressives, all the patients taking amitriptyline, but only half those receiving zimelidine gained weight (Coppen *et al.*, 1979). Such findings would suggest that both ciclazindol and zimelidine justify further evaluation in the long-term management of depressed obese patients.

## OBESITY-RELATED HYPERTENSION

The evidence linking hypertension to obesity is impressive and the management of the obese hypertensive must include weight control because this alone will reduce the blood pressure even in the normotensive (Jung et al., 1979a). For every kg of weight loss, a fall in blood pressure of approximately 3–2 mg/Hg can be expected (Reisein et al., 1978; Ramsay et al., 1978). Inability to lose weight may necessitate the introduction of, or increase in, hypotensive therapy. It is theoretically possible that the use of beta adrenergic blocking drugs may adversely influence the potential for weight loss. Conversely, the sympathomimetic anti-obesity agents may potentiate the pressor effects of catecholamines and antagonize the adrenergic neuron-blocking drugs such as bethanidine and debrisoquine. A number of studies have assessed the effects of appetite suppressants with hypertension.

Mazindol 2 mg/day for 12 weeks resulted in an additional mean weight loss of 2.0 kg and a mean reduction in systolic and diastolic blood pressure of 3 mg/Hg and 4 mg/Hg respectively when compared with placebo (Adams, 1975). In an 8-week study, diethylpropion achieved a mean weight loss of 6 kg and a reduction in mean systolic and diastolic blood pressures of 12% and 4% respectively, whereas the mean weight changes in the placebo group were 3.8 kg and 7% and 4% in systolic and diastolic pressures (Evanselista, 1968). With both drugs, it seems probable that any improvement in blood pressure control can be attributed to the additional weight loss achieved (Follows, 1971; Seedat and Reddy, 1974; Mabadeje and Johnson, 1978), so it is not surprising that mazindol and diethylpropion have comparable effects on blood pressure (Murphy et al., 1975; General Practitioner Research Group, 1978).

In contrast, fenfluramine appears to enhance rather than antagonize the effects of hypotensive therapy (Pinder et al., 1975). The effects are most marked in patients taking methyldopa and reserpine while those on debrisoquine show minimal change (Waal-Manning and Simpson, 1969). Conversely, weight losses are reduced in patients taking fenfluramine along with hypotensive agents, other than diuretics. In one 8-week study of obese hypertensives, the mean weight losses achieved with fenfluramine 60 mg/day and diethylpropion 75 mg/day were comparable and trivial (1.6 kg and 1.5 kg respectively). There was a significant difference in the change in blood pressure, falling by a mean of 16/17 mg/Hg on fenfluramine compared with 2 − +2 on diethylpropion (Follows, 1971).

In a long-term study, 96 obese hypertensives and 80 normotensives were treated with fenfluramine 80 mg/day for a year (Table X) (Hudson, 1977). The greatest reduction in blood pressure occurred during the initial 4 weeks of therapy at a time when there was little difference in the rate of weight reduction between patients receiving fenfluramine compared with placebo. The evidence would therefore suggest that while the reduction in blood pressure is partly related to weight loss, fenfluramine exerts a significant and independent hypotensive effect. It is difficult to explain the degree of the rise of systolic blood pressure that occurred in the normotensive patients when the drug was discontinued. There is an additional justification for considering long-term fenfluramine therapy in the obese hypertensive.

*Table X.* Efficacy of prolonged fenfluramine therapy in obese hypertensives on a modified Marriott diet.

| Groups (number) | Weight change (kg) | | | Change in B.P. (mmHg) systolic/diastolic | | |
|---|---|---|---|---|---|---|
| | 1/12 | 6/12 | 6/12 off therapy | 1/12 | 6/12 | 6/12 off therapy |
| [a] Control diet alone (15) | −3.6 | −6.2 | — | −11/4 | −15/6 | — |
| [b] Normotensive (80) | −4.2 | −9.8 | +6.2 | −19/10 | −19/13 | +42/17 |
| [b] Hypertensive (96) | −4.4 | −10.5 | +6.2 | −29/16 | −35/20 | +26/14 |

[a] Including some mild hypertensives.     [b] Given fenfluramine 80–120 mg daily.
(Derived from Hudson 1977.)

## OBESITY AND DIABETES

Although the exact nature of the relationship remains unclear, obesity and diabetes mellitus are frequently associated (West and Kalbleisch, 1971). Maturity onset diabetes accounts for at least 80% of the diabetic population. Of such patients, 75% are overweight. The functional pancreatic beta cell mass of obese diabetics is inadequate only in relation to body weight. Reduction in weight will improve glucose tolerance and may restore elevated insulin secretion rates to normal (Keen *et al.*, 1978). Conversely, poor dietary and diabetic control may accelerate the development of non-specific large vessel complications (Goldner *et al.*, 1971, Jarrett and Keen, 1975). It follows that there are additional reasons for achieving permanent weight loss in the obese diabetic. Unfortunately, the long-term results of dietary restriction are disappointing, and only the minority will achieve an acceptable weight.

In a third or more, diet alone will fail to control the symptoms of diabetes and hypoglycaemic therapy may be required. A sulphonylurea compound is often effective though weight gain is common during such treatment. In the already overweight, increasing obesity is highly undesirable and constitutes a major drawback to treatment with either insulin or a sulphonylurea. It follows that a particularly strong case could be made for the use of anti-obesity agents in the management of the overweight diabetic. The administration of either phentermine or diethylpropion to obese diabetics for a period of up to 24 weeks, has been shown to increase weight loss without adversely affecting glucose tolerance (Fineberg, 1961; Silverstone and Buckle, 1966; Williams, 1968; Campbell *et al.*, 1977; Gershberg, 1977) though disappointingly, the degree of weight loss may be less marked in patients already receiving biguanide.

Claims have been made that both fenfluramine and mazindol have effects

on carbohydrate and fat metabolism over and above the benefits attributable
to weight reduction. The acute administration of oral mazindol impairs
glucose absorption from the small bowel and *in vitro* increases peripheral
glucose utilization (Harrison *et al.*, 1975: Kirby and Turner, 1977). It can be
given with safety to obese diabetics (Saunders and Breidahl, 1976: Slama *et al.*,
1978). However, in such patients, the mean additional weight loss achieved
during 12 weeks of mazindol therapy was disappointing (1.4 kg) and was not
associated with any significant improvement in glucose tolerance (Bandisode
and Boshell, 1975). It would appear that mazindol is comparable in this
respect to phentermine and diethylpropion.

The metabolic effects unrelated to weight loss which have been attributed to
fenfluramine, include the inhibition of lipogenesis in adipose tissue and an
insulin dependent increase in peripheral glucose utilization (Turner, 1978).
However, studies of the metabolic effect of fenfluramine in the obese *non*-
diabetic have failed to show any significant difference in glucose tolerance,
plasma lipids and plasma insulin (Garrow *et al.*, 1972: Petrie *et al.*, 1975). In
contrast, studies of up to 6 months duration in maturity onset obese diabetics,
have reported improvement of glucose tolerance which can be only partly
related to weight loss (Dykes, 1973; Luntz and Reuter, 1975; Kesson and
Ireland, 1976; Doar *et al.*, 1979; Wales, 1979). Possibly, these conflicting
findings may reflect a greater degree of hyperinsulinaemia in the obese non-
diabetic.

At present, the evidence would suggest that fenfluramine may prove a useful
alternative to biguanide in the management of dietary resistant maturity onset
diabetes, particularly in those in whom obesity is a greater problem than
diabetes. Pending the results of further long-term studies, it might be
advisable to restrict its use to those who are intolerant or unresponsive to metformin.

## The Biguanides

Despite nearly 25 years of clinical use, the mode of action of the biguanides
remains uncertain. They have no effect on the pancreatic beta cell. They may
reduce energy intake by a central action (Patel and Stowers, 1964; Stowers and
Bewsher, 1969), delay gastric emptying (Gomez-Perez *et al.*, 1974), impair the
uptake of nutrients from the small bowel (Czyzyk, 1969), reduce gluconeo-
genesis and lipogenesis (Sterne, 1964; Muntoni, 1974) and enhance peripheral
glucose utilization (Butterfield and Whichelow, 1962). Both phenformin and
metformin are well absorbed. Metformin is excreted unchanged in the urine;
phenformin is partly metabolized in the liver, only 50% being excreted unchanged by the kidneys. Following oral administration, peak levels occur
within 3 h and the plasma half-life is approximately 11 h (Mehnert, 1969;
Alkalay, 1975).

The common side-effects include anorexia, nausea and metallic taste, vomiting and diarrhoea. The incidence is often dose-related and can be minimized
by starting with a small dose taken with meals and gradually increasing.

Biguanides have fibrinolytic effects and caution is necessary during concomitant anticoagulant therapy (Hamblin, 1971). The most serious side-effect is lactic acidosis. This is particularly likely to occur with phenformin, may arise spontaneously, and carries a high mortality (Alberti and Nattrass, 1977). Because of this, metformin is the biguanide of choice. Metformin related lactic-acidosis is associated with renal, cardiac or hepatic insufficiency. The drug should not be given to patients with such conditions and should be withdrawn during any intercurrent illness which may precipitate circulatory failure or tissue hypoxia.

Contrary to the findings of the University Group Diabetes Programme (Knatterud et al., 1975) long-term studies in the UK have failed to show any significant harmful effect of the biguanides on cardiovascular morbidity or mortality in diabetes (Keen, 1975). Unlike the sulphonylureas, the biguanides will improve diabetic control without producing weight gain. Indeed, they may promote weight loss given alone (Mirsky and Schwartz 1966; Lavieuville and Isnard, 1975; Cairns et al., 1977) or with a sulphonylurea (Patel and Stowers, 1964).

Two cross-over studies have compared treatment with metformin for 1 year with chlorpropamide for 1 year in the non-obese and obese poorly controlled insulin dependent diabetic. In both studies, the drugs produced comparable improvement in diabetic control but there were significant differences in weight change, mainly due to weight gain with the sulphonylurea. In the non-obese, metformin produced a mean weight loss of 1.5 kg compared with a mean weight gain of 4.6 kg with chlorpropamide (Clarke and Campbell, 1977). In the obese, the mean weight loss with metformin was 1.2 kg and the mean weight gain with chlorpropamide was 5.2 kg (Clarke and Duncan, 1968). Clearly, increasing obesity in poorly controlled diabetes is undesirable, and in such patients, metformin is a safe and effective adjunct to dietary therapy. At present, this comprises the most obvious example of the justification of long-term drug therapy albeit that the anti-obesity effect is secondary to the hypoglycaemic action.

## UNCONVENTIONAL PHARMACOLOGICAL APPROACHES

### Biguanides in the Non-Diabetic

Various studies have failed to show any significant weight loss with biguanides in the non-diabetic and it has been suggested that they are only effective in diabetes or possibly in patients with a family history of diabetes (Roginsky and Barnett, 1966; Faludi et al., 1968: Pearson and Mather, 1969; Hart and Cohen, 1970). However, when given double-blind to non-diabetic patients with refractory obesity, the mean additional weight loss of 0.3 kg/week (Munro et al., 1969) compares favourably with that achieved by other drugs (Table V), though a direct comparison showed metformin to be less effective than fenfluramine and more likely to cause side-effects (Lawson *et al.*, 1970). Possibly, metformin is only effective when the dosage is increased to the maximum tolerable. Its role in the management of the non-diabetic remains controversial.

## Human Chorionic Gonadotrophin (HCG)

The use of HCG in obesity was first suggested following the observation that it produced changes in appetite and body configuration without weight change in patients with Frohlich's syndrome (Simeons, 1954). It has been claimed that it will enhance well-being during severe calorie deprivation and may prevent subsequent weight regain (Simeons, 1964; Asher and Harper, 1973; Bradley, 1977). In one study, the results were quite exceptional (Politzer *et al.*, 1963). Twenty grossly obese outpatients were treated with regular HCG injections during 28 weeks of severe calorie restriction producing a mean weight loss of 41 kg. When reviewed 1 year later, all but two were said to have maintained their weight loss. Double-blind studies however have failed to demonstrate any advantage of HCG over placebo (Bray and Greenway, 1976). Currently, there is no accepted place for HCG in the treatment of obesity.

## L-dopa and Bromocriptine

Both L-dopa and bromocriptine have dopaminergic properties. In animals, L-dopa suppresses food intake (Leibowitz, 1978). In Parkinsons disease, it reduces hunger and may produce weight loss (Thompson *et al.*, 1970: Vardi *et al.*, 1976). In obesity, it prevents the fall in resting metabolic rate normally associated with dietary restriction (Shetty *et al.*, 1979). Bromocriptine, an ergot derivative, inhibits the catabolism of dopamine (Calne *et al.*, 1976). In the non-obese, it increases plasma growth hormone levels but it does not correct the abnormally low plasma growth hormone levels observed in obesity (Harrower *et al.*, 1979). These subjects appear to have a defective hypothalamic response to L-dopa stimulation, and it has been suggested that they may also have a glucoreceptor sensitivity leading to the hyperinsulinism of obesity (Laurian *et al.*, 1975). However, the administration of L-dopa to a maximum dose of 4.8 g daily failed to produce weight loss during a 6-month double-blind study in the obese (Quaade *et al.*, 1974). Similarly, bromocriptine failed to induce weight loss when given without dietary restriction (Harrower *et al.*, 1977). In both studies, anorexia and nausea were frequently observed though body weight, and presumably food intake, were unaffected. It would therefore seem that neither are of value in the management of obesity.

## Gamma-linolenic Acid

The prostaglandins are synthesized from essential fatty acids including linolenic acid. This is physiologically inactive until converted into the prostaglandin precursor gamma-linolenic acid. In the "developed countries", in spite of an adequate intake of polyunsaturated fats, a relative gamma-linolenic acid deficiency may be common because its formation is impaired by a high fat or high carbohydrate diet, in diabetes and in the elderly (Bremner, 1971).

It has been suggested that the prostaglandins and their precursors may influence the development of obesity by virtue of their regulatory effect on lipid metabolism and insulin activity (Horrobin *et al.*, 1979). Evening Primrose Oil is the richest natural source of essential fatty acids. When given in a daily dose of 2–4 g (180–360 mg of gamma linolenic acid) for 6–8 weeks, 16 subjects, 10% or more in excess of their standard weight, lost a mean of 4.1 kg, whereas none of 22 non-obese subjects lost weight (Vaddadi and Horrobin, 1979). The possibility that gamma-linolenic acid may have weight-reducing properties merits further evaluation.

## THE USE OF THYROID HORMONES ON OBESITY

### Introduction

Resting metabolic activity accounts for a considerable proportion of total energy expenditure especially during the thermogenic response to food and following environmental change (Hoffman *et al.*, 1979). There is increasing evidence to suggest that one of the major problems facing the overweight is a reduction in this metabolic activity (Miller and Parsonage, 1975; Sims, 1976). This can be illustrated by a difference in response to noradrenaline infusion (Jung *et al.*, 1979b) and may be related to a relative deficiency of metabolically active brown adipose tissue (Rothwell and Stock, 1979). Whatever the explanation, such patients are less likely to benefit from a drug which influences appetite than from one which promotes thermogenesis or energy expenditure in some other manner.

Although tests of thyroid function are normal in most obese subjects (Strata *et al.*, 1978) radio-iodine studies of triiodothyronine ($T_3$) and thyroxine ($T_4$) in the obese have shown a shortened plasma half-life (Benoit and Durrance, 1965; Rabinowitz and Myerson, 1967). In some substantially obese patients, the TSH response to TRH is exaggerated and it seems possible that their thyroid gland is relatively unresponsive to TSH (Schmitt *et al.*, 1977; Ford *et al*, 1980). Adaptive changes in thyroid hormone metabolism occur during dietary restriction. Reduction in carbohydrate intake will increase the hepatic conversion of $T_4$ to reverse $T_3$ which is physiologically inactive. This results in the "low $T_3$ syndrome" with apparently normal thyroid function and no change in the total serum thyroxine (Portnay *et al.*, 1973; Danforth *et al.*, 1978). The use of thyroid hormones in obesity is therefore the subject of continuing interest.

### Clinical Pharmacology

$T_3$ and $T_4$ are well absorbed from the small intestine. Circulating $T_4$ is almost completely protein-bound and has a biological potency one fifth that of $T_3$.

Approximately 40% of $T_4$ is converted in the liver to $T_3$. The plasma half-life of $T_3$ and $T_4$ are 2 and 7 days respectively.

Thyroid hormones increase the activity of membrane-bound ATPase, mitochondrial glycerol phosphate dehydrogenase and DNA transcription resulting in an increase in resting metabolic rate, decreased lipogenesis and increased protein turnover. The weight loss following thyroid hormone therapy is principally the result of protein catabolism. The negative nitrogen balance persists for at least 4 weeks and probably longer though it can be minimized either by increasing dietary protein or the use of anabolic steroids and growth hormone.

Common symptoms of toxicity include nervousness, excessive perspiration, palpitations, tiredness and diarrhoea. More serious long-term adverse effects include cardiomyopathy and diabetes mellitus. Thyroid hormone should be used with caution in patients with hypertension or ischaemic heart disease. In addition, because of protein binding, there is a mutual drug interaction when used concomitantly with digoxin, warfarin, tricyclic anti-depressants, aspirin and phenytoin.

## Clinical Efficacy

Both $T_3$ and $T_4$ given in pharmacological doses appear to be well tolerated by the obese. A number of studies have confirmed that the thyroid hormones will promote weight loss when given during semi-starvation (Moore *et al.*, in press), conventional dietary restriction (Hollingsworth *et al.*, 1970; Gonzalez-Barranco *et al.*, 1973) or without dietary advice (Gwinup and Poucher, 1967). They even enhance the weight loss achieved by amphetamine (Kaplan and Jose, 1970). Mean weight regain is the rule when treatment is discontinued (Gwinup and Poucher, 1967). The long-term follow-up of patients previously treated with $T_3$ suggests that these results are no different to those achieved by conventional dietary restriction (Glennon, 1966; Goodman, 1969). Because of the inherent dangers of long-term therapy and the lack of permanent weight loss with short-term administration, we would advise that the use of thyroid hormones should be restricted at present to that small but well-defined group of obese patients in whom metabolic studies suggest a degree of subclinical hypothyroidism. However, it seems possible that the future pharmacological treatment of obesity may well depend upon the development of drugs that enhance thermogenesis.

## SUMMARY

(1) The risks of drug misuse and dependency associated with amphetamine and phenmetrazine are such that they should not be prescribed as appetite suppressants. Caution should be exercised in the use of other anorectic drugs particularly if there is a previous history of drug misuse, drug dependence or psychiatric illness.

(2) Since anorectic drugs do not help to establish a new and permanent eating habit, they should only be prescribed as part of an overall management plan including appropriate dietary advice with behavioural modifications.

(3) Phentermine, diethylpropion, mazindol and fenfluramine will all produce an additional mean rate of weight loss of approximately 0.2 kg/week. These drugs are of comparable efficacy but none is free from side-effects. With the exception of fenfluramine, they are best given intermittently on the grounds of efficacy, safety and cost benefit.

(4) The individual response to drug therapy is extremely variable and may reflect differences in the metabolic adaptations which occur in obesity as much as individual susceptibilities to drug tolerance.

(5) Following drug withdrawal, weight regain is the rule. It follows that the use of anorectic drugs for up to 6 months can only be justified in selected patients with significant obesity in whom there is a well defined short-term objective.

(6) Prolonged therapy may be justified in some patients whose obesity or obesity-related disease poses a considerable threat to their physical or mental well-being. However, the long-term use of antiobesity drugs cannot be generally recommended until it has been evaluated further.

(7) The depressed, the hypertensive or the diabetic with a weight problem, require special consideration.

(8) The biguanides have a weight-stabilizing effect in poorly controlled diabetes. Metformin would appear to be the drug of first choice for this group.

(9) The indications for the pharmacological treatment of obesity remain poorly defined at present. A number of new approaches are being evaluated and it may be that future progress lies in the development of drugs which enhance thermogenesis, and thereby increase energy expenditure, rather than reduce energy intake, or in drugs which act on the peripheral mechanisms concerned in the regulation of feeding behaviour (see Chapter 1).

## REFERENCES

Adams, V. J. (1975). The efficacy and safety of Sanorex (mazindol) in exogenous obese hypertensive patients. *In* "Recent Advances in Obesity Research I" (A. Howard, ed.) pp. 393–395, Newman Publishing Ltd, London.

Alberti, K. G. M. M. and Nattrass, M. (1977). Lactic acidosis. *Lancet* ii, 25–29.

Alfaro, R. D., Gracanin, V. and Schlueter, E. (1960). A clinical pharmacologic evaluation of diethylpropion. *J. Lancet* (USA) 80, 526–530.

Alkalay, D. (1975). Pharmacokinetics of phenformin in man. *J. Clin. Pharmacol.* 15, 446.

Allen, G. S. (1975). A practical regimen for weight reduction in family practice. *J. Int. Med. Res.* 3, 40–44.

Ascher, W. L. and Harper, H. W. (1973). Effect of human chorionic gonadotrophin on weight loss, hunger and feeling of well-being. *Am. J. Clin. Nutrition* 26, 211.

Ashwell, M. A. (1973). A survey of patients' views on doctors' treatment of obesity. *Practitioner* 211, 653.

Bandisode, M. S. and Boschell, B. R. (1975). Double-blind clinical evaluation of mazindol (42–548) in obese diabetics. *Curr. Therap. Res.* **18**, 816.

Beckett, A. H. (1979). A comparative study of the pharmacokinetics of fenfluramine, ethylamphetamine, diethylpropion and their metabolites. *Curr. Med. Res. &Opinion* **6**, suppl. 1, 107–117.

Benoit, F. L. and Durrance, F. Y. (1965). Radiothyroxine turnover in obesity. *Am. J. Med. Sci.* **249**, 647.

Berchtold, P., Berger, M., Greiser, E., Dohse, M., Irmscherk, K., Gries, F. A. and Zimmerman, M. (1977). Cardiovascular risk factors in gross obesity. *Int. J. Obesity* **1**, 219.

Blundell, J. E., Latham, C. J., Moniz, E., McArthur, R. A. and Rogers, P. J. (1979). Structural analysis of the actions of amphetamine and fenfluramine on food intake and feeding behaviour in animals and in man. *Curr. Med. Res. & Opinion* **6**, suppl. 1, 34–54.

Bolodeoku, J. A., Adadeuch, B. K. and Palmer, E. O. (1972). Therapeutic effect of fenfluramine (ponderax) in obese Nigerians—weight reducing and hypotensive properties. *Nigerian Med. J.* **2**, 199.

Bradley, P. J. (1977). Human chorionic gonadotrophin in weight reduction. *Am. J. Clin. Nutrition* **30**, 649.

Bray, G. A. and Greenway, F. L. (1976). Pharmacological approaches to treating the obese patient. *In* "Clinics in Endocrinology & Metabolism" Vol. 5, No. 2. 455 (M. J. Albrink, ed.), W. B. Saunders & Co. Ltd., London, Philadelphia and Toronto.

Bremner, R. R. (1971). The desaturation step in the animal biosynthesis of polyunsaturated fatty acids. *Lipids* **6**, 567.

Brightwell, D. R. and Naylor, C. S. (1979). Effects of a combined behavioural and pharmacologic program on weight loss. *Int. J. Obesity* **3**, 141–145.

Butterfield, W. J. H. and Whichelow, M. J. (1962). The hypoglycaemic action of phenformin. Effect of phenformin on glucose metabolism in peripheral tissues. *Diabetes* **II**, 281.

Cairns, A., Shalet, S., Marshall, A. J. and Hartog, M. (1977). A comparison of phenformin and metformin in the treatment of maturity-onset obese diabetics. *Diabète et Métabolisme* **3**, 183.

Calne, D. B., Kartzinel, R. and Shoulson, I. (1976). An ergot derivative in the treatment of phentermine in obese diabetic patients. *Practitioner* **218**, 851.

Cambell, C. J., Bhalla, I. P., Steel, J. M. and Duncan, L. J. P. (1977). A controlled trial of phentermine in obese diabetic patients. *Practitioner* **218**, 851.

Campbell, D. B. (1971). Plasma concentration of fenfluramine and its metabolite, norfenfluramine, following single and repeated oral administration. *Brit. J. Pharmacol.* **43**, 465.

Carabillo, E. A. (1978). U.S.A. Drug Abuse warning network. *In* "Central Mechanism of Anorectic Drugs", (S. Garattini and R. Samanin, eds) ,p. 461. Raven Press, New York.

Carney, D. E. and Tweddell, E. D. (1975). Double-blind evaluation of long acting diethylpropion hydrochloride in obese patients from a general practice. *Med. J. Aust.* **1**, 13–15.

Clarke, B. F. and Campbell, I. W. (1977). Comparison of metformin and chlorpropamide in non-obese maturity-onset diabetics uncontrolled by diet. *B.M.J.* **2**, 1576.

Clarke, B. F. and Duncan, L. J. P. (1968). Comparison of chlorpropamide and metformin treatment on weight and blood glucose response of uncontrolled obese diabetics. *Lancet* **i**, 123.

Cohen, S. (1977). Diethylpropion (tenuate): An infrequently abused anorectic. *Psychosomatics* **18**, 28.

Connell, P. H. (1975). Central nervous system stimulation. *In* "Meylers Side Effects of Drugs", (M. N. G. Dukes, ed.), Vol. 8, 1. Excerpta Medica, Amsterdam and Oxford.

Conte, A. (1973). Evaluation of Sanorex—a new appetite suppressant. *Obesity & Bariatric Med.* **2**, 104.

Coppen, A., Rama Rao, V. A., Swade, C. and Wook, K. (1979). Zimelidine: A therapeutic and pharmacokinetic study in depression. *Psychopharmacology* **63**, 199.

Craddock, D. (1973). "Obesity & its Management". Churchill Livingstone, London and New York.

Csillag, E. R. (1971). Stimulant drugs — their use and misuse. *Med. J. Aust.* **968.**

Czyzyk, A. (1969). Impairment of intestinal glucose absorption by biguanide derivatives. *Acta. Diab. Lat.* **62**, suppl. 1, 636.

Danforth, E., Burger, A. G., Goldman, R. F. and Sims, E. A. H. (1978). Thermogenesis during weight gain. *In* "Recent Advances in Obesity Research II" G. A. Bray, p. 229. ed. Newman Publishing Ltd, London.

Doar, J. W. H., Thomson, M. E., Wilde, C. E. and Sewell, P. F. J. (1979). The influence of fenfluramine on oral glucose tolerance tests, plasma sugar and insulin levels in newly-diagnosed late-onset diabetic patients. *Curr. Med. Res. & Opinion* **6**, suppl. 1. 247–254.

Duncan, L. J. P., Rose, K. and Meiklejohn, A. P. (1960). Phenmetrazine hydrochloride and methylcellulose in the treatment of refractory obesity. *Lancet* i, 1262.

Dykes, J. R. W. (1973). The effect of a low calorie diet with and without fenfluramine on the glucose tolerance and insulin secretion of obese, maturity-onset diabetics. *Postgrad. Med. J.* **49**, 318.

Editorial. *Med. J. Austr.* (1970). Diethylpropion psychosis. p. 1052.

Enzi, G., Baritussio, A., Machion, E. and Crepaldi, G. (1976). Short-term and long-term clinical evaluation of a non-amphetamine anorexiant (mazindol) in the treatment of obesity. *J. Int. Med. Res.* **4**, 305.

Evans, J. (1959). Psychosis and addiction to phenmetrazine (Preludin) *Lancet* ii, 152.

Evanselista, I. (1978). Management of the over-weight patient with cardiovascular disease: double-blind evaluation of an anorectic drug, diethylpropion hydrochloride. *Curr. Therap. Res.* **10**, 217.

Faludi, G., Chayes, Z. and Gerber, P. (1968). Rational treatment of the obese diabetic. *Postgrad. Med. J.* **43**, 92.

Fineberg, S. K. (1961). Obesity, diabetes and anorexigenics. *J. Am. Med. Assoc.* **175**, 680.

Fink, M., Shapiro, D. M. and Itil, T. N. (1971). EEG profiles of fenfluramine, amobarbital and dextroamphetamine in normal volunteers. *Psychopharmacol.* **22**, 369.

Fletcher, L., Torosdag, A. and Bryant, J. M. (1961). Studies of the effects of phenmetrazine (Preludin) in cardiovascular disease. *Amer. J. Med. Sci.* **241**, 491.

Follows, O. J. (1971). A comparative trial of fenfluramine and diethylpropion in obese, hypertensive patients. *Brit. J. Clin. Pract.* **25**, 236.

Ford, M. J., Cameron, E. H. D., Ratcliffe, J. G., Horn, D. B., Toft, A. D. and Munro, J. F. (1980). TSH response to TRH in substantial obesity. *Int. J. Obesity* **4**, 121.

Gagnon, M. A., Bordileau, J. W. and Tetreault, L. (1969). Fenfluramine: study of its central action through its effects on sleep. *Int. J. Clin. Pharmacol.* **1**, 74.

Garrow, J. S. (1978). *In* "Energy Balance and Obesity in Man", Second Edition. North Holland Publishing Co., Amsterdam.

Garrow, J. S. (1979). Weight penalties. *B.M.J.* **2**, 1171.

Garrow, J. S., Belton, E. A. and Daniels, A. (1972). A controlled investigation of the 'glycolyptic' action of fenfluramine. *Lancet* **ii**, 559.

General Practitioner Research Group (1978). Clinical trials: comparative merits of two weight reducing drugs. *J. Pharmacotherapy* **1**, 35.

Gersberg, H., Kane, R., Hulse, M. and Phensgen, E. (1977). Effects of diet and an anorectic drug (phentermine resin) in obese diabetics. *Curr. Therapeutic Res.* **22**, 814.

Ghose, K., Rama Rao, V. A., Bailey, J. and Coppen, A. (1978). Antidepressant activity and pharmacological interaction of ciclazindol. *Psychopharmacology* **57**, 109.

Glennon, J. A. (1966). Weight reduction — an enigma. *Arch. Inter. Med.* **118**, 1.

Gogerty, J. H., Honlitan, W., Galen, M., Eden, P. and Penberthy, C. (1968). Neuropharmacological studies on an imidaze-isoindole derivative. *Fed. Proc.* **27**, 501.

Goldner, M. F., Knatterud, G. L. and Prout, T. E. (1971). The University Group Diabetes Program. Effects of hypoglycaemic agents on vascular complications in patients with adult-onset diabetes. *J. Am. Med. Assoc.* **218**, 1400.

Gomez, G. (1975). Obese patients in general practice: a comparison of the anorectic effects of mazindol, fenfluramine and placebo. *Clin. Trials J.* **12**, 38.

Gomez-Perez, F. J., Ryan, J. R. and Staub, B. (1974). Influence of pehnformin on gastric emptying rate. *J. Clin. Pharmacol.* **14**, 261.

Goodman, N. G. (1969). Triiodothyronine and placebo in the treatment of obesity. *Med. Ann. Dis. of Columbia* **38**, 658–662.

Gonzalez-Barranco, J., Schulte, J., Rull, J. A. and Lozano-Castaned, O. (1975). Triiodothyronine -v- placebo in obesity. Double-blind cross-over study. *In* "Recent Advances in Obesity Research: I" (A. Howard, ed.), p. 386. Newman Publishing Ltd, London.

Greenbaum, R. A. (1979). Ciclazindol: An adjunct to weight control. *J. Pharmacotherapy* (in press).

Gunnar Gotestam, K. (1979). A behavioural and pharmacological treatment for obesity with a 3-year follow-up. *Curr. Med. Res. & Opinion* **6**, suppl. 1, 255–259.

Gwinup, G. and Poucher, R. (1967). A conrolled study of thyroid analogs in the therapy of obesity. *Am. J. Med. Sci.* **254**, 416–420.

Hadler, A. J. (1972). Mazindol, a new non-amphetamine anorexigenic agent. *J. Clin. Pharmacol.* **12**, 453–458.

Hamblin, T. J. (1971). Interaction between warfarin and phenformin. *Lancet* **ii**, 1323.

Harrison, L. C., King-Roach, A. P. and Sandy, K. C. (1975). Effects of mazindol on carbohydrate and insulin metabolism in obesity. *Metabolism* **24**, 1353.

Harrower, A. D. B., Yap, P. L., Nairn, I. M., Walton, H. J., Strang, J. A. and Craig, A. (1977). Growth hormone, insulin and prolactin secretion in anorexia nervosa and obesity during bromocriptine treatment. *B.M.J.* **2**, 156.

Hart, A. and Cohen, H. (1970). Treatment of obese non-diabetic patients with phenformin. A double-blind cross-over trial. *B.M.J.* **1**, 22–24.

Haugen, H. N. (1975). Double-blind cross-over study of a new appetite suppressant. *Eur. J. Clin. Pharmacol.* **8**, 71.

Hinsvark, O. N., Truant, A. P., Jenden, D. J. and Steinburn, J. A. (1973). The oral bioavailability and pharmacokinetics of soluble and resin-bound forms of amphetamine and phentermine in man. *J. Pharmacokin. & Biopharm.* **1**, 319.

Hoekenga, M. J., Dillon, R. H. and Leyland, H. M. (1978). A comprehensive review of diethylpropion hydrochloride. *In* "Central Mechanisms of Anorectic Drugs" (S. Garattini and R. Samanin, eds), p. 391. Raven Press, New York.

Hoffman, M., Pfeifer, W. A., Gundlach, B. L., Nikrake, H. G. M., Oude Ophius,

A. J. M. and Hantvast, J. G. A. J. (1979). Resting metabolic rate in obese and normal weight women. *Int. J. Obesity* **3**, 111.

Innes, J. A., Watson, M. L., Ford, M. J., Munro, J. F., Stoddart, M. E. and Campbell, D. B. (1977). Plasma fenfluramine levels, weight loss and side effects. *B.M.J.* **2**, 1322.

Isbell, H. and Chrusciel, T. L. (1970). Dependence liability of "non-narcotic" drugs. *Bulletin W.H.O.*, Suppl. to Vol. 43, 66.

Hollingsworth, D. R., Amatruda, T. T. and Scheig, R. (1970). Quantitative and qualitative effects of triiodothyronine in massive obesity. *Metabolism* **19**, 934.

Horrobin, D. R., Oka, M. and Manku, M. S. (1979). Regulation of prostaglandin E 1 formation: A candidate for one of the fundamental mechanisms involved in the action of Vitamin C. *Medical Hypotheses* **5**, 849.

Hudson, K. D. (1977). The anorectic and hypotensive effect of fenfluramine in obesity. *J. Roy. Coll. Gen. Pract.* **27**, 497.

James, W. P. T., Davies, H. L., Bailes, J. and Dauncey, M. J. (1978). Elevated metabolic rates in obesity. *Lancet* **i**, 1122.

Jarrett, R. J. and Keen, H. (1975). Diabetes and athersclerosis. *In* "Complications of Diabetes" (H. Keen and R. J. Jarrett, eds), p. 179. Arnold, London.

Jasinski, D. R., Nutt, J. G. and Griffith, J. D. (1974). Effects of diethylpropion and d-amphetamine after subcutaneous and oral administration. *Clin. Pharmacol. Ther.* **16**, 645.

Jung, R. T., Shetty, P. S., Barrand, M., Callingham, B. A. and James, W. P. T. (1979a). The role of catecholamines in hypotensive response to dieting. *B.M.J.* **1**, 12.

Jung, R. T., Shetty, P. S., James, W. P. T., Barrand, M. A. and Callingham, B. A. (1979b). Reduced thermogenesis in obesity. *Nature*, **279**, 322–323.

Kaplan, N. W. and Jose, A. (1970). Thyroid as an adjuvant to amphetamine therapy of obesity. A controlled double-blind study. *Am. J. Med. Sci.* **260**, 105–111.

Keen, H. (1975). Antidiabetic agents and vascular events. *J. Clin. Path* **28**, suppl. 99.

Keen, H., Thomas, B. J., Jarrett, R. J. and Fuller, J. F. (1978). Nutritional factors in diabetes mellitus. *In* "Diet of Man: Needs & Wants". (J. Yudkin, ed.), p. 89. Applied Science; London.

Kesson, C. M. and Ireland, J. T. (1976). Phenformin compared with fenfluramine in the treatment of obese diabetic patients. *Practitioner* **216**, 577.

Kirby, M. J. and Turner, P. (1977). Ciclazindol and mazindol on glucose uptake into human isolated skeletal muscle: no interaction of mazindol with methysergide. *Brit. J. Clin. Pharmacol.* **4**, 459.

Knatterud, G. L., Meinert, C. L., Klimt, C. R., Osborne, R. K. and Martin, D. B. (1975). The U.G.D.P.: A study of the effects of hypoglycaemic agents on vascular complications in patients with adult-onset diabetes—Evaluation of phenformin therapy. *Diabetes* **24**, suppl. 1, 65.

Krotkiewski, M., Sjostrom, L., Bjorntorp, P., Carlgren, G., Carellick, G. and Smith, U. (1977). Adipose tissue cellularity in relation to prognosis for weight reduction. *Int. J. Obesity* **1**, 395.

Langlois, K. J., Forbes, J. A., Bell, G. W. and Grant, G. F. (1974). A double-blind clinical evaluation of the safety and efficacy of phentermine hydrochloride (Fastin) in the treatment of exogenous obesity. *Curr. Therap. Res.* **16**, 289–296.

Lasagna, L. (1973). Attitude towards appetite suppressants. *J. Am. Med. Assoc.* **225**, 44.

Laurian, L., Ayalon, D., Oberman, Z., Cordova, T., Horer, E., Herzberg, M. and Harell, A. (1975). Under-responsiveness of obese subjects to l-dopa stimulation. *In*

"Recent Advances in Obesity Research: I Proceedings of the First International Congress on Obesity" (A. Howard, ed.), p. 407. Newman Publishing Ltd, London.

Lavieuville, M. and Isnard, F. (1975). Retrospective study of the cardiovascular fate of 190 diabetics treated for five years or more with diguanides alone. *Journées de Diabétalogie Hôtel Dieu* **341**.

Lawson, A. A. H., Strong, J. A., Roscoe, P. and Gibson, A. (1970). Comparison of fenfluramine and metformin in the treatment of obesity. *Lancet* i, 437–441.

Leibowitz, S. F. (1978). Identification of catecholamine receptor mechanisms in the perifornical lateral hypothalamus and their role in mediating amphetamine and L-dopa anorexia. *In* "Central Mechanisms of Anorectic Drugs" (S. Garattini and R. Samanin, eds), p. 39. Raven Press, New York.

Le Riche, H. (1960). A study of appetite suppressants in general practice. *Canad. Med. Assoc. J.* **82**, 467.

Le Riche, W. H. and Csima, A. (1967). A long acting appetite suppressant drug. *Canad. Med. Assoc. J.* **97**, 1016.

Levin, A. (1975). The non-medical use of fenfluramine by drug dependent young South Africans. *Postgrad. Med. J.* suppl. 1, **183**.

Levine, S. (1979). A controlled comparative trial of a new anti-depressant—Ciclazindol. *J. Int. Med. Res.* **7**, 1.

London, A. M. and Schreiber, E. D. (1966). A control study of the effects of group discussion of anorexiants in out patient treatment of obesity with attention to the psychological aspects of dieting. *Ann. Int. Med* **65**, 80–92.

Luntz, G. R. W. N. and Reuter, C. J. (1975). A six month study of a carbohydrate restricted diet in the management of maturity-onset diabetes and an evaluation of fenfluramine in patients unresponsive to this diet. *Postgrad. Med. J.* **51**, suppl. 1, 133.

Mabadeje, A. F. B. and Johnson, T. O. (1978). A double-blind cross-over clinical trial of mazindol in obese Nigerians. *Curr. Therap. Res.* **24**, 534.

Maclay, W. P. and Wallace, M. G. (1977). A multicentre general practice trial of mazindol in the treatment of obesity. *Practitioner* **218**, 431.

McQuarrie, H. G. D. (1975). Clinical assessment of the use of an anorectic drug in a total weight reduction program. *Curr. Therap. Res.* **17**, 437–443.

Matthews, P. A. (1975). Diethylpropion in the treatment of obese patients seen in general practice. *Curr. Therap. Res* **17**, 340–346.

Mehnert, H. (1969). Pharmocokinetics of blood glucose lowering biguanide derivatives. *Acta. Diab. Lat.* **62**, suppl. 1, 137.

Miach, P. J., Thomson, W., Doyle, A. E. and Levis, W. J. (1976). Double-blind cross-over evaluation of mazindol in the treatment of obese hypertensive patients. *Med. J. Aust.* **2**, 378.

Miller, D. S. and Parsonage, S. (1975). Resistance to slimming. Adaptation or illusion. *Lancet* i, 773.

MIMS (1979). Monthly Index of Medical Specialities. Haymarket Publishing Ltd, London. Vol. 21 **10**, 169.

Mirsky, S. and Schwartz, M. (1966). Phenformin diabetic control and body weight. *J. Mount Sinai Hosp.* **33**, 180.

Moore, R., Grant, A. M. and Howard, A. N. The treatment of obesity with triiodothyronine in conjunction with a very low calorie liquid formula diet. *Int. J. Obesity* (in press).

Morselli, P. L., Maggini, C., Placidi, G. F., Gemeni, R. and Tegneni, G. (1978). An integrated approach to the clinical pharmacology of anorectic drugs. *In* "Central Mechanisms of Anorectic Drugs" (S. Garattini and R. Samanin, eds), p. 243. Raven Press, New York.

Munro, J. F., MacCuish, A. C., Marshall, A., Wilson, E. M. and Duncan, L. J. P. (1969). Weight reducing effect of biguanides on obese non-diabetic women. *B.M.J.* 2, 13.

Munro, J. F., MacCuish, A. C., Wilson, E. M. and Duncan, L. J. P. (1968). Comparison of continuous and intermittent anorectic therapy in obesity. *B.M.J.* 1, 352.

Munro, J. F., Seaton, D. A. and Duncan, L. J. P. (1966). Treatment of refractory obesity with fenfluramine. *B.M.J.* 2, 624–625.

Muntoni, S. (1974). Inhibition of fatty acid oxidation by biguanides: Implications for metabolic physiopathology. *In* "Advances in Lipid Research: Vol. 12" (Paoletti *et al.*, eds), p. 311 Academic Press, London and New York.

Murphy, J. E. Donald, J. F., Molla, A. A. and Crowder, D. (1975). A comparison of mazindol (Teronac) with diethylpropion in the treatment of exogenous obesity. *J. Int. Med. Res.* 3, 202.

Noble, R. E. (1971). A controlled study of a weight reduction regimen. *Curr. Therap. Res.* 13, 685.

Nolan, G. R. (1975). Use of anorexic drug in a total weight reduction program in private practice. *Curr. Therap. Res.* 18, 332.

Opitz, K. (1978). Tolerance and cross-tolerance to the anorexigenic effect of appetite suppressants in rats. *Int. J. Obesity* 2, 59.

Patel, D. P., and Stowers, J. M. (1964). Phenformin in weight reduction of obese diabetics. *Lancet* i, 282.

Pearson, A. M. and Mather, H. G. (1969). Phenformin as an aid to weight reduction. *Br. J. Clin. Pract.* 23, 336.

Petrie, J. C., Mowat, J. A., Bewsher, P. D. and Stowers, J. M. (1975). Metabolic effects of fenfluramine—a double-blind study. *Postgrad. Med. J.* 51, suppl. 1, 139.

Pinder, R. M., Brogden, R. N., Sawyer, P. R., Speight, T. M. and Avery, G. S. (1975). Fenfluramine: a review of its pharmacological properties and therapeutic efficacy in obesity. *Drugs* 10, 241.

Poindexter, A. (1960). Appetite suppressant drugs: a controlled clinical comparison of benzphetamine, phenmetrazine, d-amphetamine and placebo. *Curr. Therap. Res* 2, 354.

Politzer, W. M., Bershon, I. and Flaks, J. (1963). Biochemical changes resulting from drastic weight loss in obesity. *S. Afr. Med. J.* 37, 151.

Portnay, G. I., O'Brian, J. T., Bush, J., Vageriakis, A. G., Azizi, F., Arky, R., Ingbar, S. H. and Braverman, L. E. (1973). Effects of prolonged starvation on serum TSH, $T_4$ and $T_3$ concentration in man. *Clin. Research* 2, 958.

Printzmetal, M. and Alles, G. A. (1940). The central nervous stimulant effects of dextro-amphetamine sulphate. *Amer. J. Med. Sci.* 200, 665.

Quaade, F., Pakkenberg, H. and Juhl, E. (1974). Levodopa as a treatment of obesity. *Acta. Med. Scand.* 195, 129.

Rabinowitz, J. L. and Myersen, R. M. (1967). The effects of triiodothyronine in some metabolic parameters of obese individuals. Blood $\vartheta\rho CO\sigma$, the biological life of T$\delta$ and the concentration of T$\delta$ on adipose tissue. *Metabolism* 16, 68.

Ramsay, L. E., Ramsay, M. H., Hettiarachchi, J., Davies, D. L. and Winchester, J. (1978). Weight reduction in a blood pressure clinic. *B.M.J.* 2, 244.

Reisin, E., Abel, R., Modan, M., Silverberg, D. S. Eliahou, H. and Modan, B. (1978). Effect of weight loss without salt restriction on the reduction of blood pressure in overweight hypertensive patients. *New Eng. J. Med.* 298, 1.

Roginsky, M. S. and Barnett, J. (1966). Double-blind study of phenethyldiguanide in weight control of obese non-diabetic subjects. *Am. J. Clin. Med.* 19, 223.

Rothwell, N. J. and Stock, M. J. (1979). A role for brown adipose tissue in diet-induced thermogenesis. *Nature* 281, 31.

Sandoz Pharmaceuticals (1973). Sanorex. A monograph. Sandoz INC New Jersey.

Saunders, M. and Breidahl, H. (1976). The effect of an anorectic agent (mazindol) on control of obese diabetics. *Med. J. Aust.* **2**, 576.

Schapiro, M. M. and Brogan, N. (1960). Dietless weight loss with benzphetamine (Didrex): a controlled comparison with phenmetrazine and placebo. *Curr. Therap. Res.* **2**, 333.

Schmitt, T., Lugman, W., McCool, C., Lenz, F., Ahmad, U., Nolan, S., Stephen, T., Sunder, J. H. and Danowski, T. S. (1977). Unresponsiveness to exogenous TSH in obesity. *Int. J. Obesity* **1**, 185–190.

Scoville, B. A. (1973). Review of amphetamine-like drugs by the Food and Drug Administration: Clinical data and value judgements. *In* "Obesity in Perpective" Proceedings of the Fogarty Conference (G. A. Bray, ed.) p. 441. Washington. U.S. Government.

Seaton, D. A., Duncan, L. J. P., Rose, K. and Scott, A. M. (1961). Diethylpropion in the treatment of refractory obesity. *B.M.J.* **1**, 1009.

Seaton, D. A., Rose, J. and Duncan, L. J. P. (1964). A comparison of the appetite suppressing properties of dexamphetamine and phentermine. *Scot. Med. J.* **9**, 482.

Seedat, Y. K. and Reddy, J. (1974). Diethylpropion hydrochloride (Tenuate Dospan) in the treatment of obese hypertensive patients. *S. Ar. Med. J.* **48**, 569.

Shetty, P. S., Jung, R. T. and James, W. P. T. (1979). Effect of replacement with levodopa on the metabolic response to semi-starvation. *Lancet* **i**, 77–79.

Silverstone, J. T. (1974). Intermittent treatment with anorectic drugs. *Practitioner* **213**, 245–252.

Silverstone, J. T. and Buckle, R. M. (1966). Obesity in diabetes. Some considerations of treatment. *Am. J. Clin. Nutrition* **19**, 158.

Silverstone, J. T. and Lascelles, B. D. (1965). A double-blind trial of durophet-M in the treatment of obesity in general practice. *J. Roy. Coll. Gen. Pract.* **9**, 304.

Simeons, A. T. W. (1954). The action of chorionic gonadotrophin in the obese. *Lancet* **ii**, 946.

Simeons, A. T. M. (1964). Chorionic gonadotrophin in the treatment of obesity. *Am. J. Clin. Nutrition* **15**, 188.

Sims, E. A. H. (1976). Experimental obesity, dietary-induced thermogenesis and their clinical implications. *In* "Clinics in Endocrinology and Metabolism" (M. J. Albrink, ed.), Vol. 5, No. 2, p. 377. W. B. Saunders & Co. Ltd, London, Philadelphia and Toronto.

Slama, G., Selmi, A., Hautecouverture, M. and Tchobroutsky, G. (1978). Doubleblind dietical trial of mazindol on weight loss, blood glucose, plasma insulin and serum lipids in overweight, diabetic patients. *Diabète et Métabolisme* **4**, 193.

Smith, R. C. F. (1962). The long term control of obesity using sustained release appetite suppression. *Brit. J. Clin. Pract.* **16**, 6.

Smith, R. G., Innes, J. A. and Munro, J. F. (1975). Double-blind evaluation of mazindol in refractory obesity. *B.M.J.* **3**, 284.

Spillane, J. P. (1960). The use of phenmetrazine. *Practitioner* **185**, 102.

Steel, J. M. and Briggs, W. (1972). Withdrawal depression in obese patients after fenfluramine treatment. *B.M.J.* **3**,. 26.

Steel, J. M., Munro, J. F. and Duncan, L. J. P. (1973). A comparative trial of different regimens of fenfluramine and phentermine in obesity. *Practitioner* **211**, 232–236.

Sterne, J. (1964). The present state of knowledge on the mode of action of the antidiabetic guanides. *Metabolism* **13**, 791.

Stowers, J. M. and Bewsher, P. D. (1969). Studies on the mechanism of weight reduction by phenformin. *Postgrad. Med. J.* **45**, suppl. 1, 13.

Strata, A., Ugolotti, G., Contini, C., Magnati, G., Pugnoli, C., Tirelli, F. and Zuliani, U. (1978). Thyroid and obesity: survey of some function tests in a large obese population. *Int. J. Obesity* **2**, 333.

Stunkard, A. S. and Brownell, K. D. (1979). Behaviour therapy and self-help programmes for obesity. *In* "The Treatment of Obesity" (Current Status of Modern Therapy, Vol. 2) (J. F. Munro, ed.), p. 199. MTP Press Ltd, Lancaster.

Thomson, R. A., White, J. E. and Echols, E. L. (1970). The effect of L-dopa therapy in Parkinson's disease. *Arizone Med.* **27**, 5.

Truant, A. P., Olon, L. P. and Cobb, S. (1972). Phentermine resin as an adjunct in medical weight reduction: a controlled, randomised double-blind prospective study. *Curr. Therap. Res.* **14**, 726–738.

Turner, P. (1978). How do anti-obesity drugs work. *Int. J. Obesity* **2**, 343.

Turner, P. (1979). Peripheral mechanism of action of fenfluramine. *Curr. Med. Res. & Opinion* **6**, suppl. 1, 101.

Vaddadi, K. S. and Horrobin, D. F. (1979). Weight loss produced by Evening Primrose Oil administration in normal and schizophrenic individuals. *I.R.C.S. Med. Sci.* **7**, 52.

Vardi, J., Oberman, Z., Rabey, I., Streifler, M., Ayalow, D. and Herzberg, M. (1976). Weight loss in patients treated with levodopa. *J. Neurol. Sci.* **30**, 33.

Vernace, B. J. (1974). Controlled comparative investigations of mazindol, D-amphetamine and placebo. *Obesity & Bariatric Med.* **3**, 124.

Waal-Manning, H. J. and Simpson, F. O. (1969). Fenfluramine in obese patients on various antihypertensive drugs. Double-blind controlled trial. *Lancet* **ii**, 1392.

Wales, J. K. (1979). The effect of fenfluramine on obese, maturity-onset diabetic patients. *Curr. Med. Res. & Opinion*, **6**, suppl. 1, 226.

Wallace, A. G. (1976). AN 448 Sandoz (Mazindol) in the treatment of obesity. *Med. J. Aust.* **1**, 343.

West, K. M. and Kalbleisch, J. M. (1971). Influence of nutritional factors on the prevalence of diabetes mellitus. *Diabetes* **20**, 99.

"Which? Way to Slim" (1978). Consumers' Assoc. (Edith Rudinger, ed.) Eyre, & Spottiswoode Ltd, Portsmouth.

Williams, J. (1968). Trial of a long-acting preparation of Diethylpropion in obese diabetics. *Practitioner* **200**, 411.

Wing, R. R. and Jeffrey, R. W. (1979). Out-patient treatments of obesity: a comparison of methodology and clinical results. *Int. J. Obesity* **3**, 261.

Wright, G. J., Lang, J. F., Lemieux, R. E. and Goodfriend, M. J. (1975). The objective and timing of drug disposition studies. Appendix III. Diethylpropion and its metabolites in the blood plasma of the human after subcutaneous and oral administration. *Drug. Metab. Review* **4**, 267.

Yelnosky, J. O. and Lawlor, R. B. (1970). A comparative study of the pharmacologic actions of amphetamine and fenfluramine. *Arch. Int. Pharmacodyn* **184**, 374.

Yelnosky, J. O., Panasevich, R. E., Borrelli, A. R. and Lawlor, R. B. (1969). Pharmacology of phentermine. *Arch. Int. Pharmacodyn* **178**, 62.

# 7 □ Drug Treatment of Anorexic States

## G. I. Szmukler

Every variety of treatment has been given these patients, limited only by the preconceptions and ingenuity of the Physician, and the availability of pharmacological agents. Each procedure has initially received enthusiastic support and has achieved successes as well as abysmal failures.

Bliss and Branch (1960) *Anorexia Nervosa*

Anorexia and disturbances of eating are common symptoms in psychiatric practice. While this chapter will concentrate on the treatment of anorexia nervosa, a condition which can be reliably differentiated from other psychological disorders associated with eating problems, a brief review of these other conditions will be presented first.

## ANOREXIA AND EATING DISORDERS IN MENTAL ILLNESS

Surprisingly little attention has been given to a consideration of the pathogenesis of disorders of eating which are so common in a wide variety of mental illnesses.

Depressive illness may be associated with almost complete anorexia and emergency treatment of this disorder may be life-saving on this account. Paykel (1977) has reported on changes in appetite encountered in depression. Of his patients, 66% reported a diminution of appetite, 14% an increase and in 20%, there was no change. An enhanced appetite was almost limited to female patients with a "neurotic" rather than "psychotic" illness, and an illness with milder symptoms.

Specific treatment for anorexia in depression is not required as this symptom improves concurrently with elevation of mood. Antidepressant medication, such as the tricyclic group of drugs, is believed to act in this disorder by effects on neurotransmitter availability, particularly of noradrenaline (NA) and serotonin (5HT) (Schildkraut, 1969). Since these substances have also been implicated in the regulation of appetite in animals (to be considered later), the possibility arises that the disturbances of mood and of appetite independently reflect neurochemical changes in the limbic diencephalic regions of the brain. The patient usually experiences a loss of interest in food (among many other things), but sometimes his reluctance to eat may be explained by him as a desire to die.

Appetite is variably affected in mania and weight loss, and often seems to be related to an extreme degree of hyperactivity and restlessness, with the patient sometimes claiming to be too busy with other, more important, affairs to eat. Quite gross weight loss may be encountered in schizophrenic illnesses. The patient may again express a lack of interest in eating, but in addition, he may harbour suspicions about his food having been tampered with, or he may act on the basis of bizarre delusional beliefs concerning food, nutritional requirements or digestive processes. Treatment in these disorders is again directed towards the underlying mental illness with the phenothiazine compounds providing the most common basis of drug treatment.

Neurotic disorders may also be associated with disturbances of appetite and eating. In some patients, anxiety may be associated with autonomic effects on gastrointestinal functioning, and the patient might experience nausea, epigastric fullness, a dry mouth or no desire to eat. There is some evidence that "neurotic" patients have more food aversions, poorer appetites and fewer food preferences than, for example, patients with asthma (Wirdum and Weber, 1961). Less commonly, obsessional fears concerning food may result in weight loss. For example, a patient recently seen by the author had reduced her consumption significantly because of rituals surrounding the act of eating. She was plagued with doubts about whether she was about to swallow, and thus destroy, something "valuable" or something "which should not be eaten" and she felt compelled to check each morsel carefully. A phobic anxiety state may limit the situations in which some sufferers may eat, for example, restaurants or the company of others may be avoided. Some patients may have a fear of vomiting in front of others and this may necessitate restrictions on where and when they eat. In all of these neurotic disorders, treatment is again directed towards the underlying illness, with medication being employed to a variable degree depending on the individual patient's presentation and the nature of the disturbance. Antidepressant drugs can prove effective in some patients, but psychological forms of treatment find more common application.

## ANOREXIA NERVOSA

Bliss and Branch (1960) in their monograph on the subject, regarded the loss of 25 lb or more, if attributable to psychological causes, as a sufficient definition of the condition. This extensive definition, which would encompass cases from almost all psychiatric categories, has been strongly challenged (Russell, 1970). The argument that a distinctive syndrome exists, which is readily recognizable clinically and which, although it has a variable outcome, remains the same with each relapse, has generally been accepted. Clear-cut criteria defining the illness have been cited (Russell, 1970; Feighner *et al.*, 1972). The hope that a specific definition of the disorder would effectively direct research towards a distinctive aetiology has to some extent been vindicated with the accumulation of some evidence implicating a distinctive endocrine disturbance. The diagnostic criteria proposed by Russell are as follows:

(1) Behaviour leading to weight loss and malnutrition: carbohydrate is avoided to a relatively greater extent than other foodstuffs. Additional devices apart from abstinence may be employed by the patient in her endeavours to lose weight. These include vomiting, purgation and excessive exercise.

(2) An early onset of amenorrhoea. In about a quarter of cases, this precedes the weight loss (Kay and Leigh, 1954). This dysfunction is often very persistent, even following refeeding and weight restoration. In the male, there is a loss of potency and sexual interest.

(3) There is a characteristic and readily recognizable psychopathology. The patient has a morbid fear of becoming fat and relentlessly pursues the goal of a thin body shape. Thinness is denied even in the face of severe emaciation. This disturbance of body image assumes the form of a powerfully held overvalued idea. The patient may fear losing control over her eating, or she may feel guilty if she consumes more than a tiny portion. Preoccupations with food (e.g. its calorie content, methods of preparation) are usually strikingly evident.

It has long been recognized that a considerable proportion of patients have periods of overeating (bulimia). It has also become clearer more recently that there is a subtype or variant of this disorder in which episodes of bulimia (during which enormous quantities of food may be ingested), accompanied by self-induced vomiting, dominate the clinical picture. These patients tend to maintain a higher body weight and menstrual functioning is more likely to be preserved. The pursuit of thinness is, however, just as prominent (Russell, 1979). The prognosis tends to be poorer (Hsu *et al.*, 1979).

Anorexia nervosa usually commences in adolescence and females are much more commonly affected than males. Estimates range from 15:1 to 5:2, females to males (Crisp and Toms, 1972; Kendall *et al.*, 1973). The illness may, however, commence at a later age and sometimes, for example, it may occur during the puerperium.

The condition is more common than was previously believed. Crisp *et al.* (1976) examined a school population in England and found a prevalence of anorexia nervosa in private schools of 1 in 100 girls in the 16–18 age group. The corresponding prevelance in a state comprehensive school population was only 1 in 550, confirming a social class differential. Wider population studies provide some evidence of an increasing incidence (Theander, 1970; Kendell *et al.*, 1973). The more recent tendency in our culture for a thin body shape to be viewed as the ideal one may play a role in at least initiating attempts at dieting and weight loss which may later become uncontrolled.

The outcome ranges from spontaneous recovery to death. Dally (1969) maintains that it is unusual for the illness to last less than 3 years and that hopes for recovery are slim if it has lasted for more than 7 years. Recent mortality rates range from 5% to 15% in the course of follow-up periods of 5 years or more. A number of careful follow-up studies point to a good recovery in less than half the patients with a poor outcome observed in about 20% to 30% (Theander, 1960; Morgan and Russell, 1975; Hsu et al., 1979). Outcome was assessed in terms of biological functions (weight, menstruation) and psychological adjustment. The illness is very damaging in its impact on the patient's interpersonal relationships both within the family and with her peers. Sexual feelings often give rise to particular concern and frequently tend to be denied.

## Pathogenesis

The pathogenesis of anorexia nervosa is poorly understood. A variety of aetiological factors and mechanisms have been postulated. Psychological theories based on psychoanalytic theory have been proposed (Thoma, 1967) as well as other psychodynamic views. Bruch (1965, 1974) has stressed the disturbance in the patient's accuracy of perception or cognitive interpretation of stimuli arising in her body as well as her paralysing sense of ineffectiveness as an individual. This is explained as a consequence of the child's needs in the past having been routinely subverted to the mother's sense of what was appropriate. Only through starvation can the patient achieve a special recognition and sense of mastery. Bruch also recognizes that the sufferer's experiences and perceptions are influenced by the malnutrition itself and its effects on central nervous system functions. Crisp (1965, 1967) has presented a model of the disorder which recognizes an interaction between biological and psychological influences. The efflorescence of puberty, with its spurt of growth and development of a feminine shape, especially when it occurs earlier than normally, may catch the adolescent girl at a time when she is psychologically unprepared for these changes. Starvation and the ensuing reversion to an immature body shape and amenorrhoea serve as a protection against the demands of femininity. Sexual feelings and drives are suppressed by the effects of starvation and this, in turn, provides a secondary reinforcement for perpetuating the disturbance. Rosman et al. (1977) have claimed the role of abnormal family dynamics to be the central one in an understanding of anorexia nervosa. Certain patterns of family interaction are described and the ill child is seen as stabilizing a disordered structure.

Most clinicians dealing with this disorder tend to find a consideration of most of the above influences useful in the management of individual patients. One of the psychological abnormalities described above has been the subject of quite intensive experimental investigation. This is the disturbance of body perception. Slade and Russell (1973) reported that by using a light-beam measuring device they were able to demonstrate that patients with anorexia nervosa considerably overestimated their body dimensions compared with normal controls. They were, however, as accurate in perceiving the dimensions of a control "model". This study also demonstrated that this distortion of perception lessened in severity as the patients regained weight, and that those patients with the greatest disturbance in body estimation were the ones most likely to lose weight following discharge from hospital. This pattern could thus provide the basis of a vicious cycle where malnutrition derives from an impaired body image which, in turn, generates more self-starvation. Unfortunately, these findings have not been consistently replicated (Crisp and Kalucy, 1974; Garner et al., 1976; Casper et al., 1979) but the relationship of over estimation to prognosis appears substantiated.

Most of the above considerations of pathogenesis do not immediately suggest a specific role for physical forms of treatment in anorexia nervosa. The past decade or so has, however, seen an intensive investigation of some of the biological disturbances so evident in this condition. These will now be briefly described as the later discussion of drug treatment will make reference to them.

## Hypothalamic Function in Anorexia Nervosa

Support for the notion that the hypothalamus may be disturbed in anorexia nervosa came originally from the observation that experimental lesions in animals produced disturbances which in some ways resembled those in patients with the disorder. The proximity of sites regulating feeding and sexual functions was noted (Donovan, 1970), and there were reports of hypothalamic tumours in man producing severe emaciation (Bauer, 1954; Lewin et al., 1972).

Considerable evidence has now accumulated of disturbances of a number of functions depending at least in part on hypothalamic regulation. The issue of greatest contention, however, is whether these abnormalities are in some way a primary aspect of the condition or whether they are simply the consequence of malnutrition. Sophisticated endocrine evaluations have not been performed on starved "normal" controls as a basis for comparison. Some of the changes associated with starvation and with anorexia nervosa are reviewed by Warren and Van de Wiele (1973).

Serum growth hormone (GH) levels have been found to be elevated but return rapidly to normal with a raised calorie intake. Findings concerning GH responses to a glucose load and to L-dopa stimulation are not consistent and it is claimed that refeeding may not so readily re-establish normal functioning (Garfinkel et al., 1975; Brown et al., 1977; Sherman and Halmi, 1977).

Thyroid function is disturbed in a manner consistent with many chronic illnesses, with low $T^3$ and $T^4$ levels. The former rises more rapidly with weight gain. Thyroid stimulating hormone (TSH) levels are normal but some patients may show a delayed response to thyrotrophin-releasing hormone (TRH) (Wakeling et al., 1979).

Abnormalities of water regulation (Russell and Bruce, 1966; Mecklenburg et al., 1974) have also been described as well as impairments in temperature regulation (Wakeling and Russell, 1970; Mecklenburg et al., 1974). These disturbances are believed to be the result of malnutrition with substantial recovery occurring as weight is regained.

The most substantial evidence linking anorexia nervosa to a hypothalamic disturbance, not readily explicable in terms of malnutrition, relates to changes in sex hormone regulation. As previously stated, amenorrhoea may precede significant weight loss. Many investigators have confirmed a significant failure in the output of the gonadotrophins LH (luteinizing hormone) and FSH (follicle-stimulating hormone) (Russell *et al.*, 1965; Wakeling, *et al.*, 1977). These hormones are regulated by gonadotrophin-releasing hormones (GnRH) from the hypothalamus and, in turn, regulate oestrogen secretion. The latter exerts negative and positive feedback effects on the hypothalamus and pituitary. As the patient's weight is restored to normal, previously low or undetectable levels of LH and FSH rise. However, not infrequently, normal weight fails to be associated with a return of menstruation and re-establishment of a normal cyclical pattern of LH release. At low weights, the action of clomiphene, which blocks the negative feedback action of oestrogen at the hypothalamus, is impaired and there is little rise of LH; this however, improves with weight gain, although even then some patients may continue to fail to respond normally (Marshall and Russell Fraser, 1971; Beumont *et al.*, 1973; Wakeling *et al.*, 1976).

The response of LH to gonadotrophin-releasing hormone (GnRH) is also impaired with emaciation but again improves with normalization of weight (Palmer *et al.*, 1975; Sherman and Halmi, 1977). In the emaciated state, the pattern of response is reminiscent of that in the prepubertal girl. It has also been observed that administration of GnRH for 3–5 days results in a restoration to normal of LH response, suggesting that pituitary capacity is preserved and that hypothalamic failure is primarily responsible (Nillius and Wide, 1975; Yoshimoto *et al.*, 1975). Finally, Wakeling *et al.* (1977) have investigated the role of oestrogen in the regulation of menstruation in patients with anorexia nervosa. In normal cycles, oestrogen has both a negative and positive feedback effect at a hypothalamic level. The latter action results in the mid-cycle surge of LH associated with ovulation. A course of ethinyl oestradiol given to patients with anorexia nervosa indicated a failure of this mechanism. With the achievement of normal weight it was re-established in a small proportion of patients at an early stage, and in nearly all eventually if their weight was maintained.

The conclusion may be drawn from these findings that there is a persistent abnormality in hypothalamic function in patients with anorexia nervosa which cannot readily be explained on the basis of weight loss and the effects of malnutrition. It should be added, however, that such studies have not been performed on "normal" malnourished females, particularly with severe emaciation and of long duration. The starvation in anorexia nervosa is also of a particular kind, with carbohydrates being particularly avoided.

Russell (1970) suggested that despite the profound psychological disturbances evident in anorexia nervosa, particularly the irrational fear of fatness which seems to explain the patient's avoidance of food, a primary hypothalamic disturbance cannot necessarily be ruled out. The observed hypothalamic dysfunction may derive from higher functional disturbances (e.g. involving the limbic system), which are perhaps impossible to disentangle from their phsychological correlates. Other possibilities include damage caused by the malnutrition itself or, alternatively, that the physiological changes and the psychopathological features are relatively independent manifestations of a primary hypothalamic defect (Mecklenburg *et al.*, 1974). These considerations are taken further by Russell (1977) who presents a model which emphasizes possible circular interactions between the psychological disorder, the endocrine disturbances and the malnutrition.

## Neurochemical Disturbances in Anorexia Nervosa

A number of reviews have been published of possible biochemical abnormalities relevant to anorexia nervosa. They are essentially based on studies of regulatory mechanisms controlling feeding in animals and the possible contribution of putative neurotransmitters to these functions. There are major limitations, however, to the conclusions which can be drawn. There is no guarantee that mechanisms found to be operative in some animals apply also to humans and in any case, a full and coherent model of feeding regulation animals has not been formulated (see Chapter 1). Problems arise when the observation of aphagia in animals is correlated with the disturbance of food intake found in anorexia nervosa. In fact, the term "anorexia" in these patients is a misnomer. Appetite is not usually impaired, and hunger continues to be perceived (Garfinkel, 1974). Some patients do deny feeling any hunger at all (Silverstone and Russell, 1967) but they are in a minority. Moreover, patients are often preoccupied with thoughts of food.

It has been argued that anorexia nervosa represents a disorder not of hunger but of satiety. Patients often say they feel "full" or "bloated" after small amounts of food. However, in addition to the problem of the elusiveness of the concept of satiety (McHugh and Moran, 1977), is the need to explain the observations that many patients have bulimic episodes in which enormous quantities of food are ingested and also of the ability of hospitalized patients to eat normal meals when supervised. Recently however, Garfinkel *et al.* (1979) have reported on differences between patients with anorexia nervosa and controls on a "satiety aversion to sucrose test". Normals rate the taste of sucrose solutions as aversive or unpleasant after ingesting a glucose load. Anorexia nervosa patients did not experience any difference in the rated pleasantness after, compared with before, glucose ingestion. This characteristic was stable for a small series of patients over a period of a year and persisted despite changes in weight.

Mawson (1974) has reviewed hypothalamic and neurotransmitter regulatory mechanisms of feeding and their implications for the treatment of anorexia nervosa. Evidence based on selective lesions in the hypothalamus and related areas and intraventricular injections of various neurotransmitters and their antagonists, is quoted in support of the hypothesis that feeding, among other activities, is mediated by noradrenergic (NA) and dopaminergic (DA) systems, while behaviour associated with satiety are mediated by cholinergic systems. "Oscillations" and "compensations" in this system, he suggests, may account for the bulimic episodes. He recognizes that DA and NA depletion in animals is usually associated with hypoactivity, while patients with anorexia nervosa remain remarkably active. The actions of amphetamines and of chlor-promazine are discussed but not readily integrated into the hypothesis. A trial of levodopa (L-Dopa) which would increase central DA is suggested.

Redmond *et al.* (1977) describe the results of locus ceruleus destruction in monkeys. This is a noradrenergic nucleus. Marked hyperphagia and hyper-dipsia result; the amount of weight gain is proportional to the reduction in the NA metabolite MHPG (3-methoxy-4-hydroxy-phenethyleneglycol) concen-trations in the nucleus' projection areas in the brain. They hypothesize that anorexia nervosa may be due to an overactivity of a NA-mediated "satiety centre" and suggest a trial of a noradrenergic blocking agent.

Another review by Barry and Klawans (1976) concludes with an hypothesis quite at variance with the one proposed by Mawson. These authors address themselves more fully to the psychopathological disturbances in anorexia nervosa, as well as the hyperactivity, sexual disturbances, age of onset, greater female incidence and the potential reversibility of the illness. A case is pre-sented for anorexia nervosa being associated with dopaminergic hyperactivity.

Evidence is cited for the following observations: a reduction of food intake in animals follows DA stimulation (e.g. amphetamines, apomorphine) and can be blocked by DA receptor antagonists (e.g. pimozide) but see Chapter 5 for studies with pimozide in man. Prolonged DA receptor stimulation in man may cause anorexia and weight loss (e.g. with L-Dopa). Chlorpromazine (a DA antagonist) results in weight gain. There is evidence that DA, in addition to regulating prolactin release, may also be involved in regulating the ovulatory LH surge but not the tonic release of LH in rats. A variety of dopaminergic agonists in rats (including bromocriptine) may block ovulation, and this may in turn be antagonized by a DA blocker. Sexual receptivity in ovariectomized rats may also be enhanced or reduced by neuropharmacological manipulation of DA. Some evidence is also discussed for the production of hypothermia by DA agonists. The psychopathological changes are linked by the authors to the disturbances of perception and thinking which have been well established as occurring in amphetamine-induced psychoses. Body image disturbances, hy-peractivity, stereotyped and compulsive behaviours and changes in libido have all been observed. Finally, the onset around puberty and the increased inci-dence in females is attributed to the major central nervous system regulatory changes occurring at this time of life and to the greater complexity of these systems in females. The greater the complexity, it is argued, the greater the risk of something going amiss. Reversibility is accounted for by a delayed establishment of feedback control which can, with time, become adequate. A DA-blocking agent, such as pimozide, would theoretically be appropriate for treatment, but the authors argue that its effect may be only temporary as more DA may be produced by a poorly controlled system.

Young (1975) has postulated that anorexia nervosa is based on an hyper-sensitivity of the hypothalamus to oestrogens. This represents a failure of maturation as the prepubertal brain shows a similar hypersensitivity. Young cites evidence that feeding is diminished in rats treated with oestrogens while hyperactivity and thermoregulatory disturbances have also been observed. Low LH levels and amenorrhoea are produced and GH levels rise. In humans, a presumed oestrogen/progestogen imbalance in favour of the former may be associated with altered emotional states and abnormal bodily sensations, particularly a feeling of being "bloated". Treatment of anorexia nervosa with progesterone is suggested as this antagonizes some of the effects of oestrogen.

The hypotheses described above present more or less plausible mechanisms for some of the features seen in anorexia nervosa. For the clinician, however, they do not seem to do justice to the experiences described by his patients (Crisp, 1978). Animal models may seem difficult to reconcile with a patient's explanation of her stubborn refusal to eat as being the result of a deliberate and purposeful quest to be thin. The need to be thin appears to override the desire for food, which may often be quite overwhelming.

Strategies for verifying these hypotheses are difficult to devise and knowledge of the neuropharmacology of drugs used in experiments is often incomplete. Their actions are unlikely to be entirely specific. There is also evidence that the constitution of the diet itself may affect the concentration of important neurochemicals. For example, 5HT levels in the brains of rats have been shown to rise following a carbohydrate-rich meal, and this process is believed to be mediated by effects on blood tryptophan levels relative to other amino acids and their availability for CNS uptake (Wurtman and Fernstrom, 1976). The diet is usually very disordered in patients with anorexia nervosa and deficiencies are somewhat selective.

Although the hypotheses presented are far from complete, they do provide a framework in which drug treatment may find a meaning. However, the question of whether any drug treatment is effective in anorexia nervosa needs to be tested empirically quite apart from any theoretical considerations.

## The Evaluation of Drug Treatment in Anorexia Nervosa

A number of considerations need to be borne in mind when treatment in anorexia nervosa is evaluated. A "good" outcome, in a condition as multifarious in its clinical manifestations as anorexia nervosa, is not simple to define. Disturbances are evident in a number of areas: behaviour directed towards food avoidance and disposal, profound psychopathological changes, disruption of endocrine status and usually a damaging effect on interpersonal and social relationships. These disturbances do not necessarily improve in parallel with treatment. An improvement in a patient's mental status or reversion to normal menstrual cycles is far from an invariable concomitant of weight gain, for example. Evaluation of outcome needs to take some account of each of these diverse areas of functioning.

Anorexia nervosa is capable of being rigorously defined and the diagnostic criteria which have been used must be clearly stated in any treatment trial. The illness is one in which the course varies between spontaneous remission and chronic disability. A control group is thus essential. Characteristics known to influence prognosis (e.g. age at onset, duration of illness, premorbid adjustment, bulimia and vomiting, etc.) must be, as far as is possible, equally represented in both treatment and comparison groups. Selection factors must be examined: for example, patients referred to a general physician may be quite different on a number of characteristics to those who find their way to a psychiatrist.

As the illness is usually a chronic one, outcome in the long term, as well as the short term, should be assessed. The goals may be quite different, with weight restoration and improvement in physiological status being the immediate aims with the prevention of future relapse and amelioration of psychosocial disabilities being those for the longer term. When the effect of medication on long-term outcome is assessed, the possibility of the drug's contribution being obscured by the impacts of life's numerous vicissitudes needs to be considered.

Finally, the treatment itself needs to be defined adequately. In addition to drug therapy, a whole array of other "treatments" are likely to be in operation. These may include separation from a disturbing family environment by admission to hospital, persuasion to eat, and non-specific nursing care. The impact on this illness in the short term at least, of hospital admission and well-organized nursing care cannot be over-emphasized. Russell (1973, 1977b) has described the results of this treatment with severely ill patients who, on admission, averaged 63% of their healthy body weight. Patients were admitted to hospital, and within one to two weeks, were consuming 3000–5000 cal/day. The nursing care was characterized by attempts to form a trusting relationship with the patient, a communication to the patient that her fears were understood, reassurance and careful supervision. The last involved certain restrictions on the patient's movements and an insistence on supervised meals so that the patients were unable to dispose of food, induce vomiting or resort to any other subterfuges aimed at producing weight loss. In this setting, patients showed themselves quite able to allow the nurses to exercise control over their eating and they were able to achieve weight gains of 200–400 g daily with a steeper rise in the early stages due to selective body retention of water. By discharge, they had achieved a mean of 84% of their healthy body weight but about 40% of the patients still experienced some resistance to food intake. These results need to be borne in mind when an uncontrolled evaluation of a drug in the treatment of anorexia nervosa is reported, and it is clear that only a properly controlled trial can take account of these non-specific treatment effects.

Such considerations indicate that an outcome study in anorexia nervosa is a difficult undertaking, and that unfortunately to date, most studies of drug treatment for this illness have failed to meet even minimal requirements to permit a reasonable evaluation.

## Chlorpromazine

Dally and Sargent (1960) were the first to advocate the use of chlorpromazine in anorexia nervosa. They also reported a follow-up of their patients 5 years later (Dally and Sargent, 1966). Chlorpromazine in doses of 300–1600 mg/day was combined with insulin. The latter was given 1 h before meals in a dose (usually 40-60 units) sufficient to make the patient sweat and become drowsy. A diet, steadily increased from 1500 to 4000 cal/day, was also provided.

The authors were able to make a comparison between three groups of patients:

(a) Those treated with chlorpromazine and insulin (30 patients)
(b) Those treated with insulin alone (8 patients)
(c) Those who had bed rest without specific treatment (27 patients).

The average weight gain per week was significantly higher for the chlorpromazine treated group-, 2.1 kg/week, compared with 1.1 kg/week for the insulin group and 1.0 kg/week for the bed-rest group. The average total weight gain was greater (10.4 kg for the chlorpromazine group, compared with 8.1 kg and 5.4 kg), and the average time in hospital was less (36 days compared with 59 days and 44 days). The authors attributed the weight gain to the drug overcoming the patient's resistance to food and panic at the prospect of eating.

The follow-up study, however, revealed no significant differences in overall outcome between the chlorpromazine plus insulin group compared with the non-specific treatment group. Of the former, 33% and of the latter, 30% had readmission within 2 years of leaving hospital while 69% of the former and 72% of the latter were menstruating regularly 3–5 years later. Of the chlorpromazine group, 72% compared with 60% of the bed-rest group were well adjusted socially and maintained a satisfactory weight on follow-up, a non-significant difference.

A number of other findings were also of interest. Of the chlorpromazine-treated group, 30%, compared with 20% of the non-specific control group lost weight within a month of discharge. In addition, more patients from the former group developed a period of compulsive overeating (45% compared with 12%). Menstruation took almost twice as long to return, on average, in the patients treated with chlorpromazine. This was possibly an effect of the drug itself which is known sometimes to cause amenorrhoea. This careful follow-up study revealed no long-term advantages of chlorpromazine and it may indeed have been associated with some drawbacks.

Chlorpromazine is known to be associated with weight gain in patients treated for other conditions, and it is also known to have effects on neuroendocrine function. The release of FSH and LH is diminished, and temperature regulation is impaired (Byck, 1975). These changes are obviously not in the desired direction for patients with anorexia nervosa. In principle, the administration of large doses of a drug to an emaciated patient in metabolic disarray seems undesirable unless there are compelling reasons for it. Dally and Sargant reported an incidence of epileptic fits in 10% of their patients treated with chlorpromazine. Most clinicians would find this unacceptable. There have also been case reports of the occurrence of a haemolytic anaemia in anorectic patients treated with chlorpromazine (How and Davidson, 1977). From a theoretical standpoint, the dopamine antagonistic properties of the drug may have some significance (Barry and Klawans, 1976), but other actions such as noradrenergic and cholinergic blockade have also been noted.

Clinical experience indicates that there may be an occasional place for the administration of moderate doses of chlorpromazine in patients who become extremely anxious at the prospect of eating. There is no reason to believe, however, that chlorpromazine is more effective for this purpose than any other tranquillizing drug.

## Insulin

Insulin was originally introduced because of its appetite stimulant properties. Dally and Sargant (1966) showed no difference in outcome, either in the short-term or the long-term, between patients treated with insulin (without chlorpromazine) and those treated with bed rest. There is no evidence that insulin has a place in the treatment of anorexia nervosa. Not only is it dangerous for emaciated patients to be treated in this way, but its appetite-stimulating properties are unnecessary as the patients are usually already hungry or quickly become so during treatment.

## Antidepressants

Feelings of depression, guilt and anxiety are common among patients with anorexia nervosa but although they rate themselves more highly on these emotions than control subjects, they do not score as highly as patients diagnosed as depressed (Folstein et al., 1977). Suicide now ranks as the commonest cause of death in fatal cases. The relationship between anorexia nervosa and depression may be explicable in a number of possible ways. It has been argued that anorexia nervosa represents a variant of depressive illness (Cantwell et al., 1977). The age of onset, the consistency of the syndrome, both across patients and with time, and the frequent absence of symptoms typical of a depressive illness fail to support this hypothesis. King (1963) considered that a division of anorexia nervosa into "primary" and "secondary" types was justified. The former represented a specific and homogeneous syndrome while the latter was composed of a mixture of various psychiatric states (including depression) in which the anorexic component happened to occur as a pathoplastic development. Some patients with a later onset of the illness (e.g. in the puerperium) and with an atypical presentation, may be examples of the "secondary" type. An alternative explanation for the occurrence of depressive symptoms in typical cases of anorexia nervosa could be that they are a consequence of the malnutrition. The patients studied by Folstein et al. (1977), for example, showed an improvement in mood after weight gain.

Halmi et al. (1978) found that a group of patients with anorexia nervosa had significantly lower urinary levels of 3-methoxy-4-hydroxyphenylglycol (MHPG) than a control group. About 25% of MPHG is believed to derive from central nervous system noradrenaline metabolism and some patients with depressive illness are reported to have low levels. In this study, there seemed to be a relationship between MHPG and the symptoms of depression, although the patients did not qualify for a diagnosis of depression. The possibility is discussed that these patients might represent a subtype within the rubric of anorexia nervosa, and also that MHPG levels might be used as a predictor of response to antidepressant medication in this disorder. There is evidence, for example, that patients suffering from a depressive illness respond better to imipramine if urinary MHPG levels are low and better to amitriptyline if they are high (Beckmann and Goodwin, 1975).

Weight gain and carbohydrate craving are common in patients with depression on maintenance amitriptyline therapy following recovery (Paykel *et al.*, 1973). The mechanism of action is not known, but these authors speculate about an alteration in hypothalamic sensitivity to blood glucose levels. Considerations such as these provide a rationale for a treatment trial of antidepressant in anorexia nervosa.

Mills *et al.* (1973) described 80 patients with "self-starvation amenorrhoea", i.e. they had amenorrhoea of at least 6 months' duration, had made a determined effort to exclude carbohydrates from their diet and were unable voluntarily to increase their carbohydrate intake when at an obviously subnormal weight. After careful examination for the presence of depressive features, these workers claimed to find positive indications of depression in 81% of the patients. All were treated with either nortriptyline or amitriptyline. A follow-up for an undisclosed period was reported for just over half of the patients, but the results appear unexceptional and provide no evidence to support the use of this medication.

Needleman and Waber (1976, 1977) described the use of amitriptyline for six consecutive inpatients in a paediatric setting. The rationale for this treatment was stated by the authors as deriving from their observtions that many patients with anorexia nervosa display signs of "motor and speech retardation" and express feelings of sadness. All patients began to gain weight between the sixth and twelfth day of treatment, and this was preceded by a "rather striking brightening of mood", increased warmth of the extremities and noticeable improvement in social relationships. The patients' self-reported attitudes to eating were also claimed to have changed. However, as this study was uncontrolled and reported on a small number of patients with a relatively recent onset of illness, the results could have been entirely due to such non-specific factors as hospitalization, separation from the family and general nursing care.

Single case reports have appeared describing the effect of amitriptyline in patients with anorexia nervosa. Kendler (1978) argued that this drug by its action on 5HT could alter a "set-point' for weight regulation in the same way as it can alter mood "set-points". A patient with anorexia nervosa was described who became obese following treatment with amitriptyline. She was hungry all the time and could not be satiated. An analogy was drawn between this change and the switch observed in some patients with bipolar affective disorder from depression to mania when treated with amitriptyline. Moore (1977) described a patient whose bulimia and vomiting improved dramatically when amitriptyline was commenced, recurred when the drug was stopped and improved again with its re-institution.

It may be concluded that a specific role for antidepressant drugs in the treatment of this illness remains to be demonstrated, but that on the other hand, a good clinical trial has still to be conducted. An indication for the use of this type of medication still remains, however, on clinical grounds when severe depressive symptoms are present, particularly when they have failed to improve with weight restoration. The risk of suicide should be remembered. The expectation need not be held that the symptoms characteristic of anorexia nervosa will be ameliorated by this treatment, but an improvement in mood in a depressed patient may facilitate her general management.

## Cyproheptadine

Cyproheptadine (Periactin) is an antagonist of histamine and 5HT. Lavenstein *et al.* (1962) found that asthmatic children treated with cyproheptadine (as compared with another antihistamine drug, chlorpheniramine) showed weight gain, increased appetite and augmented linear growth. Noble (1969) administered the drug to 20 healthy underweight adult outpatients in a controlled double-blind study. Over the 56 days of treatment, patients on cyproheptadine gained significantly more weight and rated their appetites as significantly enhanced. Weight gain was not due to water retention or hyperadrenocorticism and fasting blood glucose levels were unaltered. Other studies on underweight (not anorexic) patients have reported similar results. (Silvert, 1971; Silverstone and Schuyler, 1975).

The use of cyproheptadine has some interest from a theoretical standpoint. There is considerable evidence from animal studies that 5HT plays a role in feeding behaviour, and that increased availability of 5HT leads to reduced eating by what appears to be a premature recognition of satiety (Barrett, 1978). However, the administration of tricyclic antidepressants such as amitriptyline, which are effective in blocking neuronal re-uptake of 5HT and thus increasing 5HT availability at receptor sites, fails to produce anorexia in man. Benady (1970) used cyproheptadine in the treatment of a 12-year-old girl described as a "classical case" of anorexia nervosa, and found it successful following previous failures with other treatments.

Two controlled trials have examined the use of this drug in patients with anorexia nervosa. Vigersky and Loriaux (1977) performed a double-blind study on 26 patients on a metabolic ward who met Feighner's criteria for diagnosis. Patients were given 12 mg/day for 8 weeks following discharge and were weighed weekly. Thirteen patients received cyproheptadine and 11 placebo. Weight gain was not significantly different for the two groups. A later comparison by the authors of the two groups of patients revealed, however, that they were not initially matched for certain variables that have been shown to be linked to prognosis: older age on onset, longer duration of illness and incidence of vomiting. Patients in whom a poorer prognosis would have been anticipated were over-represented in the cyproheptadine-treated group.

The second trial was reported by Goldberg *et al.* (1979). Eighty female patients, rigorously defined, were allocated at random to one of four treatment options: cyproheptadine (with or without behaviour therapy) *vs* placebo (with or without behaviour therapy). Drug allocation was double-blind. Dosage started at 12 mg/day and was increased by 4 mg every 5 days if the patient had failed to gain at least 0.5 kg in the intervening period, up to a maximum of 32 mg/day. Results were assessed in terms of weight gain. There was no overall difference between the cyproheptadine and placebo groups. However, the authors found a small sub-sample of patients in whom cyproheptadine seemed to induce a significantly greater weight gain. They were patients with a history of birth delivery complications or weight loss in the order of 50% from the norm, or a history of past outpatient treatment failure. The intercorrelations between these three variables were modest, indicating that a single underlying factor was unlikely. Virtually no side-effects of the drug were noted.

The evidence thus indicates that cyproheptadine fails to produce a major impact on the illness, even when weight alone forms the criterion of improvement. A few patients with severe emaciation may derive some benefit.

## Levodopa

It will be recalled that Mawson (1974) suggested a trial of L-dopa on the basis of his hypothesis that anorexia nervosa was associated with a depletion of central dopamine and/or noradrenaline.

Levodopa (L-dopa), the immediate precursor of dopamine, has found a place in the treatment of Parkinson's disease, a condition in which a relative deficiency of dopamine is implicated in the pathogenesis. Johanson and Knorr (1974, 1977) have reported on the use of L-dopa in anorexia nervosa. The authors view certain features of this illness as bearing some relationship to those seen in Parkinsonism. They describe anorexic patients as having "rigid, obsessive-compulsive, stereotyped behaviour that involves eating and movement and the development of rituals". Their experience of these patients had been of evident weakness and inactivity rather than the more commonly described hyperactivity. Most clinicians would question these observations or at least formulate them in other ways.

Nine inpatients were given L-dopa by Johanson and Knorr for 16 to 27 days in doses from 0.2 to 3.0 g/day. Five of these patients exhibited a gain of weight between 3 and 5.5 kg while in hospital. These patients were continued on L-dopa following discharge and four continued to gain weight. Several patients commented that they felt better on the medication and no severe adverse effects were noted with these comparatively low dosages.

No conclusions can be drawn from this report as it is uncontrolled and the patients treated are few. The authors' belief that L-dopa may be used with "better than average possibility of success" seems premature at this stage.

## Bromocriptine

Bromocriptine is a specific DA agonist and again, a trial of this treatment would be supported by a dopamine depletion hypothesis of anorexia nervosa. This is discussed by Harrower (1978). Dopamine depletion would be expected to result in raised blood prolactin levels as prolactin secretion is under hypothalamic control and prolactin-inhibiting factor is believed to be identical with dopamine. Some patients with secondary amenorrhoea (e.g. the amenorrhoea-galactorrhoea syndrome) have evidence of raised prolactin secretion, and menstruation has been restored in some cases with bromocriptine therapy (Williams, 1977). Most studies have shown normal levels of prolactin in anorexia nervosa (Wakeling *et al.*, 1979) but the possibility remains that separate pathways may be involved.

Harrower *et al.* (1977) reported trivial and inconsistent changes in weight in a group of eight patients with anorexia nervosa given bromocriptine for 2–4 weeks.

## Other Drugs in Anorexia Nervosa

Redmond *et al.* (1976), who have proposed an important role for noradrenaline in mediating satiety and an overactivity of this neurotransmitter in anorexia nervosa, reported a single case study of a patient treated with the α-adrenergic blocking agent, phenoxybenzamine. The patient gained weight on this drug while losing weight during a prior evaluation period of no treatment and also during a period of treatment with a β-adrenergic blocker.

Plantey (1977) reported a dramatic improvement in a patient treated with pimozide, a dopaminergic receptor blocker. This result was offered in support of Barry and Klawan's dopaminergic hyperactivity hypothesis of anorexia nervosa.

Moldofsky *et al.* (1977) provided a preliminary report on the use of meto-clopramide in five patients with anorexia nervosa. Complaints of fullness and bloating after small meals are common among patients with this disorder and these may suggest a delay in gastric emptying. Metoclopramide is an anti-emetic drug which hastens gastric emptying and relaxes the duodenal cap. The drug was administered to the five patients in a double-blind, placebo con-trolled trial over a period of 4 weeks, 2 weeks on the drug and 2 weeks on placebo in a random allocation. After each meal, patients rated symptoms of flatulent dyspepsia. The effect of the medication was favourable, and all subjects described a greater ability to finish their meals. Three patients con-tinued with the medication for 3 to 6 months with marked relief of symptoms. Weight changes were not reported, and the authors added a cautionary note that metoclopramide may affect prolactin secretion.

Tec (1971, 1977) reported on the use of nandrolone (Durabolin) in 12 patients. Effectiveness was claimed in ten cases, but few details were given.

Barcai (1977) commented on some similarities between some patients with anorexia nervosa and others with mild mania, particularly motor restlessness, impaired attention span, pressure of thought and unstable mood. Two patients, older than average, were described who responded well to lithium carbonate. In addition to feeding problems, affective-type symptoms appear to have been present. The dangers of lithium administration to patients with irregularities in weight and fluid balance were noted.

Green and Rau (1977) described four categories of compulsive eating that they could discern in 31 patients studied. They distinguished a group whom they called "True Compulsive Eaters". The characteristic features were of irregular, unpredictable episodes of bulimia during which excessively large quantities of food were ingested, as it were, against the patients' will. The experience was not associated with pleasure and anything available would be eaten. A semblance of an aura may have been reported beforehand and feelings of depersonalization were common during the episode. An abrupt termination of the episode was followed by a strong desire to go to sleep, and a short period of disorientation could be elicited if the patient was awakened. The authors considered these features to resemble some of those not uncommonly found in epileptic seizures. Five of the seven patients classified within this group had an abnormal E.E.G. and following a trial of treatment with the anti-epileptic agent, diphenylhydantoin, six showed fewer episodes of compulsive eating. Two of the patients were reported as being very thin and of actively aiming to be so.

## Inducing Menstruation

Not infrequently, patients ask if there is a way in which menstrual periods may be re-induced. Generally, they may be reassured that with a return to normal weight, periods will return spontaneously. However, as has been mentioned, there may be a considerable delay even following restoration to a normal weight. In such a case, and if there are psychological reasons for wishing an early return of menstruation, then a course of clomiphene citrate, 50–100 mg/day for 5 to 7 days may be attempted. This drug is believed to act by blocking the negative feedback action of oestrogen at the hypothalamus and results in an increase in gonadotrophin release. A menstrual period may then follow, and continuing ovulatory cycles may become re-established in some patients.

Periods may, however, be reinstated with greater certainty by the use of Luteinizing Hormone Releasing Hormone (LHRH). Nillius and Wide (1977) have reported on the induction of normal ovulatory cycles in amenorrhoeic patients with anorexia nervosa who were practically devoid of any gonadotrophic and ovarian activity before treatment. Wakeling and de Souza (unpublished data, 1980) have elaborated a regime for re-inducing periods in patients who have achieved a healthy weight. The patient is first tested for a positive feedback response of luteinizing hormone to oestrogen (100 $\mu$g orally for 3 days or, alternatively, 1 mg in ml of oestradiol benzoate injected i.m.). The positive feedback response should be apparent by the fifth day if an oral preparation is administered, or by the third day if the oestradiol is given intramuscularly. The presence of a positive response suggests an almost certain induction of menstruation with clomiphene citrate alone.

In the absence of a positive feedback response, the following regime is instituted. The patient is given clomiphene 100 mg for 7 days commencing on day 1. By day 14, the follicle should have matured and oestrogen been produced. In normal circumstances, a positive feedback response would result in a surge of LH at this stage. This LH surge is mimicked by giving LHRH 100 $\mu$g in a saline drip over a period of 5 h on day 14 when ovulation will occur in the majority of cases. These patients will then mostly go on to have regular cycles in the future.

## CONCLUSIONS

At present drug treatment plays a very minor role in the clinical management of anorexia nervosa.

The rationale for a drug treatment approach in this illness has been reviewed. The evidence for hypothalamic dysfunction is strong. Although manipulation of putative neurotransmitters such as noradrenaline, dopamine and 5HT can be shown to influence the regulation of feeding in animals, a coherent animal model appropriate to an understanding of anorexia nervosa is lacking. Hypotheses have been proposed, but these are often totally at variance with each other, are loosely supported by the evidence and fail to do justice to the complexity of the clinical picture presented by the disorder, particularly its psychopathological aspects.

Few drug trials described in the literature are sufficiently rigorous to allow firm conclusions to be drawn. Nearly all are concerned with short-term weight gain only and even then results of equal quality may be obtained by a programme relying on well organized nursing care, persuasion and a loosely psychotherapeutic approach (Russell, 1973, 1977b), or the use of a behaviourally orientated approach (Blinder et al., 1970). Results from drug treatment studies have not, in their turn, generated any biologically based hypotheses which offer the hope of an improved understanding of this illness.

A clinician reviewing studies of drug treatment in this disorder might be surprised at the absence of remarks concerning compliance with medication. If the patient is afraid of gaining weight, why should she take tablets designed to make her do so? Subterfuges are frequently resorted to in disposing of food, so one might guess the same would apply to medication. A worker, currently in the process of conducting a trial of mianserin hydrochloride at the Royal Free Hospital, while explaining the nature of a placebo-controlled trial to two patients, made the mistake of referring to the placebo as "just a sugar-coated dummy tablet". The patients became anxious and their participation was ensured only after some persuasion.

Most of the drugs tested in the treatment of anorexia nervosa have been selected because of their appetite stimulant actions. It could be argued that an appetite suppressant might be more useful in controlling what may in some cases be an enhanced appetite which the patient is constantly attempting to keep at bay. This particularly may be the case for bulimic patients. No trial of such a drug has yet been reported.

Finally, the principles of effective management of patients with anorexia nervosa have been clearly described by Russell (1973, 1977b). In the short term, hospitalization, with nursing care directed to helping the patient gain weight, usually results in a satisfactory increase. The occasional indications for the employment of chlorpromazine, antidepressants and clomiphene or LHRH have been discussed. The long-term management poses greater problems and although the emphasis has been on a psychotherapeutic approach, evidence for the effectiveness of any treatment is lacking.

## REFERENCES

Barcai, A. (1977). Lithium in adult anorexia nervosa: a pilot report on two patients. *Acta psychiatr. Scand.* **55**, 97–101.

Barrett, A. M. (1978). Neuropharmacology of appetite regulation. *Proc. nutr. Soc.* **37**, 193–199.

Barry, V. C. and Klawans, H. L. (1976). On the role of dopamine in the pathophysiology of Anorexia Nervosa. *J. neur. Transm* **38**, 107–122.

Bauer, H. G. (1954). Endocrine and other clinical manifestations of hypothalamic disease. A survey of 60 cases, with autopsies. *J. clin. Endocr. Metab.* **14**, 13.

Benady, D. R. (1970). Cyproheptadine hydrochloride (Periactin) and anorexia nervosa: A case report. *Brit. J. Psychiat.* **117**, 681–682.

Beumont, P. J. V., Carr, P. J. and Gelder, M. G. (1973). Plasma levels of luteinizing hormone and of immunoreactive oestrogens (oestradiol) in anorexia nervosa: response to clomiphene citrate. *Psychol. Med.* **3**, 495–501.

Blinder, B. J., Freeman, D. M. A. and Stunkard, A. J. (1970). Behaviour therapy of anorexia nervosa: effectiveness of activity as a reinforcer of weight gain. *Amer. J. Psychiat.* **126**, 1093–1098.

Bliss, E. L. and Branch, C. H. (1960). "Anorexia Nervosa", Paul B. Hoeber Inc., New York.

Brown, G. M., Garfinkel, P. E., Jeuniewic, N., Moldofsky, H. and Stancer, H. C. (1977). Endocrine profiles in Anorexia Nervosa. *In* "Anorexia Nervosa" (R. A. Vigersky, ed.), pp. 123–135. Raven Press, New York.

Bruch, H. (1966). Anorexia Nervosa and its differential diagnosis. *J. nerv. ment. Dis.* **141**, 555–556.

Bruch, H. (1973). "Eating Disorders". Basic Books, New York.

Byck, R. (1975). *In* "The Pharmacological Basis of Therapeutics" (Goodman and Gilman), 5th edition, p. 152. Macmillan, New York.

Cantwell, D. P., Sturzenberger, S., Burroughs, J., Salkin, B. and Green, J. K. (1977). Anorexia Nervosa: an affective disorder? *Arch. gen. Psychiat.* **34**, 1087–1093.

Casper, R. C., Halmi, K. A., Goldberg, S. C., Eckert, E. D. and Davis, J. M. (1979). Disturbances in body image estimation as related to other characteristics and outcome in anorexia nervosa. *Brit. J. Psychiat.* **134**, 60–66.

Crisp, A. H. (1965). Clinical and therapeutic aspects of anorexia nervosa—a study of 30 cases. *J. psychosom. Res.* **9**, 67–78.

Crisp, A. H. (1966). A treatment regime for anorexia nervosa. Brit. J. Psychiat., **112**, 505–512.

Crisp, A. H. and Toms, D. A. (1972). Primary anorexia nervosa or weight phobia in the male; Report on 13 cases. *Brit. med. J.* **1**, 334–338.

Crisp, A. H. and Kalucy, R. S. (1974). Aspects of the perceptual disorder in anorexia nervosa. *Brit. J. med. Psychol.* **47**, 349–361.

Crisp, A. H., Palmer, R. L. and Kalucy, R. S. (1976). How common is anorexia Nervosa? A prevalence study. *Brit. J. Psychiat.* **128**, 549–554.

Crisp. A. H. (1978). Disturbances of neurotransmitter metabolism in anorexia nervosa.

*Proc. Nutr. Soc.* **37**, 201–209.

Dally, P. G. and Sargant, W. (1960). A new treatment of anorexia nervosa. *Brit. med. J.* **1**, 1770–1773.

Dally, P. G. and Sargant, W. (1966). Treatment and outcome of anorexia nervosa. *Brit. med. J.* **2**, 793–795.

Dally, P. (1969). "Anorexia Nervosa", Heinemann Medical Books, London.

Donovan, B. T. (1970). "Mammalian Neuroendocrinology", McGraw-Hill, London.

Feighner, J. P., Robins, E., Guze, S. B., Woodruff, R. A., Winokur, G. and Munoz, R. (1972). Diagnostic criteria for use in psychiatric research. *Arch. gen. Psychiat.* **26**, 57–63.

Folstein, M. F., Wakeling, A. and DeSouza, V. (1977). Analogue scale measurement of the symptoms of patients suffering from anorexia nervosa. *In* "Anorexia Nervosa" (R. A. Vigersky, ed.), pp. 21–25. Raven Press, New York.

Garfinkel, P. E. (1974). Preception of hunger and satiety in anorexia nervosa. *Psychol. Med.* **4**, 309–315.

Garfinkel, P. E., Brown, G. M., Stancer, H. C. and Moldofsky, H. (1975). Hypothalamic-pituitary function in Anorexia Nervosa. *Arch. gen. Psychiat.* **32**, 739–744.

Garfinkel, P. E., Moldofsky, H. and Garner, D. M. (1979). The stability of perceptual disturbances in anorexia nervosa. *Psychol. Med.* **9**, 703–708.

Garner, D. M., Garfinkel, P. E., Stancer, H. C. and Moldofsky, H. (1976). Body image disturbances in Anorexia Nervosa and obesity. *Psychosom. Med.* **38**, 327–336.

Goldberg, S. C., Halmi, K. A., Eckert, E. D., Casper, R. C. and Davis, J. M. (1979). Cyproheptadine in anorexia nervosa. *Brit. J. Psychiat.* **134**, 67–70.

Green, R. S. and Rau, J. H. (1977). The use of diphenylhydantoin in compulsive eating disorders: further studies. *In* "Anorexia Nervosa" (R. A. Vigersky, ed.), pp. 337–382. Raven Press, New York.

Halmi, K. A., Dekirmenjian, H., Davis, J. M., Casper, R. and Goldberg, S. (1978). Catecholamine metabolism in anorexia nervosa. *Arch. gen. Psychiat.* **35**, 458–460.

Harrower, A. D. B., Yap, P. L., Nairn, I. M., Walton, H. J., Strong, J. A. and Craig, A. (1977). Growth hormone, insulin and prolactin secretion in anorexia nervosa and obesity during bromocriptine treatment. *Brit. med. J.* **2**, 156–159.

Harrower, A. D. (1978). Bromocriptine in anorexia nervosa. *Brit. J. hosp. Med.* **20**, 672–675.

How, J. and Davidson, R. J. (1977). Chlorpromazine induced haemolytic anaemia in anorexia nervosa. *Postgrad. med. J.* **53**, 278–279.

Hsu, L. K. G., Crisp, A. H. and Harding, B. (1979). Outcome of Anorexia Nervosa. *Lancet* **i**, 61–65.

Johanson, A. J. and Knorr, N. J. (1974). Treatment of Anorexia Nervosa by L-DOPA (letter). *Lancet* **i**, 591.

Johanson, A. J. and Knorr, N. J. (1977). L-DOPA as treatment of anorexia nervosa. *In* "Anorexia Nervosa" (R. A. Vigersky, ed.), pp. 363–372. Raven Press, New York.

Kay, D. W. and Leigh, D. A. (1954). The natural history, treatment and prognosis of anorexia nervosa based on a study of 38 patients. *J. ment. Sci.* **100**, 411–431.

Kendell, R. E., Hall, D. J., Hailey, A. and Babigan, H. M. (1973). The epidemiology of Anorexia Nervosa. *Psychol. Med.* **3**, 200–203.

Kendler, K. S. (1978). Amitriptyline-induced obesity in anorexia nervosa: a case report. *Amer. J. Psychiat* **135**, 1107–1108.

King, A. (1963). Primary and secondary anorexia nervosa syndromes. *Brit. J. Psychiat.* **109**, 470–479.

Lavenstein, A. F., Decaney, E. P., Lasagna, L. and Van Metre, T. E. (1962). Effect of cyproheptadine on asthmatic children: study of appetite, weight gain and linear growth. *J. Amer. med. Assoc.* **180,** 912–916.

Lewin, K., Mattingly, D. and Mills, R. R. (1972). Anorexia nervosa associated with hypothalamic tumour. *Brit. med. J.* **2,** 629–630.

Marshall, J. C. and Russell-Fraser, T. (1971). Amenorrhoea in anorexia nervosa: assessment and treatment with clomiphene citrate. *Brit. med. J.* **4,** 590–592.

Mawson, A. R. (1974). Anorexia nervosa and the regulation of intake: a review. *Psychological medicine* **4,** 289–308.

McHugh, P. R. and Moran, T. H. (1977). An examination of the concept of satiety in hypothalamic hyperphagia. *In* "Anorexia Nervosa" (R. A. Vigersky, ed.), pp. 67–73. Raven Press, New York.

Mecklenburg, R. S., Loriaux, D. L., Thompson, R. H., Anderson, A. E. and Lipsett, M. B. (1974). Hypothalamic dysfunction in patients with anorexia nervosa. *Medicine* **53,** 147–159.

Mills, I. H., Wilson, R. J., Eden, M. A. M. and Lines, J. G. (1973). Endocrine and social factors in self starvation amenorrhoea. *In* "Symposium—Anorexia Nervosa and Obesity" (R. F. Robertson, ed.), pp. 31–43. Royal College of Physicians, Edinburgh.

Moldofsky, H., Jeuniewic, N. and Garfinkel, P. E. (1977). Preliminary report on metoclopramide in anorexia nervosa. *In* "Anorexia Nervosa" (R. A. Vigersky, ed.), pp. 373–375, Raven Press, New York.

Moore, D. C. (1977). Amitriptyline therapy in Anorexia Nervosa. *Amer. J. Psychiat.* **134,** 1303–1304.

Morgan, H. G. and Russell, G. F. M. (1975). Value of family background and clinical features as predictors of long-term outcome in anorexia nervosa: four year follow up study of 41 patients. *Psychol. Med.* **5,** 355–371.

Needleman, H. L. and Waber, D. (1976). Amitriptyline therapy in patients with anorexia nervosa (letter) *Lancet* **ii,** 580.

Needleman, H. L. and Waber, D. (1977). The use of amitriptyline in anorexia nervosa. *In* "Anorexia Nervosa" (R. A. Vigersky, ed.), pp. 357–362. Raven Press, New York.

Nillius, S. J. and Wide, L. (1975). Gonadotrophin releasing hormone treatment for induction of follicular maturation and ovulation in amenorrhoeic women with anorexia nervosa. *Brit. med. J.* **3,** 405–408.

Nillius, S. J. and Wide, L. (1977). The pituitary responsiveness to acute and chronic administration of gonadotrophin releasing hormone in acute and recovery stages of anorexia nervosa. *In* "Anorexia Nervosa" (R. A. Vigersky, ed.), pp. 225–241. Raven Press, New York.

Noble, R. F. (1969). Effect of cyproheptadine on appetite and weight gain in adults. *J. Amer. med. Assoc.* **209,** 2054–2055.

Palmer, R. L., Crisp, A. H. Mackinnon, P. C. B., Franklin, M., Bonnar, J. and Wheeler, M. (1975). Pituitary sensitivity to 50 mg LH/FSH-RH in subjects with Anorexia Nervosa in acute and recovery stages. *Brit. med. J.* **1,** 179–182.

Paykel, E. S., Meuller, P. S., and de la Vergne, P. M. (1973). Amitriptyline, weight gain and carbohydrate craving: a side effect. *Brit. J. Psychiat.* **123,** 501–507.

Paykel, E. S. (1977). Depression and appetite. *J. Psychosomatic Research* **21,** 401–407.

Plantey, F. (1977). Pimozide in the treatment of anorexia nervosa (letter) *Lancet,* **i,** 1105.

Redmond, D. E., Huang, Y. H., Baulu, J., Snyder, D. R. and Mass, J. W. (1977). Norepinephrine and satiety in monkeys, in Anorexia Nervosa. *In* "Anorexia Nervosa" (R. A. Vigersky, ed.), pp. 81–96. Raven Press, New York.

Redmond, D. E., Swann, A. and Heninger, G. R. (1976). Phenoxybenzamine in anorexia nervosa (letter) *Lancet*, **ii**, 307

Rosman, B. L., Minuchin, S., Baker, L. and Liebman, R. (1977). A family approach to anorexia nervosa: study, treatment and outcome. *In* "Anorexia Nervosa" (R. A. Vigersky, ed.), pp. 341–348. Raven Press, New York.

Russell, G. F. M. (1970). Anorexia Nervosa: Its identity as an illness and its treatment. In "Modern Trends in Psychological Medicine: 2" (J. H. Price, ed.), pp. 131–164. Butterworth, London.

Russell, G. F. M. (1973). The management of anorexia nervosa. *In* "Symposium— Anorexia Nervosa and Obesity" (R. F. Robertson, ed.), pp. 44–62. Royal College of Physicians, Edinburgh.

Russell, G. F. M. (1977a). Editorial: The present status of anorexia nervosa. *Psychol. Med.* **7**, 363–367.

Russell, G. F. M. (1977b). General management of anorexia nervosa and difficulty in assessing the efficacy of treatment. *In* "Anorexia Nervosa" (R. A. Vigersky, ed.), pp. 277–289. Raven Press, New York.

Russell, G. (1979). Bulimia Nervosa: an ominous variant of anorexia nervosa. *Psychol. Med.* **9**, 429–448.

Russell, G. F. M. and Bruce, J. T. (1966). Impaired water diuresis in patients with anorexia nervosa. *Amer. J. Med.* **40**, 38–48.

Russell, G. F. M., Loraine, J. A., Bell, E. T. and Harkness, R. A. (1965). Gonadotrophin and oestrogen excretion in patients with anorexia nervosa. *J. Psychosom. Res.* **9**, 79–85.

Schildkraut, J. J. (1965). The catecholamine hypothesis of affective disorders: a review of supporting evidence. *Amer. J. Psychiat.* **122**, 509–522.

Sherman, B. M. and Halmi, K. A. (1977). Effect of nutritional rehabilitation on hypothalamic-pituitary function in anorexia nervosa. *In* "Anorexia Nervosa" (R. A. Vigersky, ed.), pp. 211–224, Raven Press, New York.

Silbert, M. V. (1971). The weight gain effect of periactin in anorexic patients. *S. Afr. med. J.* **45**, 374–377.

Silverstone, T. and Schuyler, D. (1975). The effect of cyproheptadine on hunger, caloric intake and body weight in man. *Psychopharm.* **40**, 335–340.

Slade, P. D. and Russell, G. F. M. (1973). Awareness of body dimension in Anorexia Nervosa. Cross-sectional and longitudinal studies. *Psychol. Med.* **3**, 188–199.

Tec. L. (1971). Anorexia Nervosa: follow up on a special method of treatment. *Amer. J. Psychiat.* **127**, 1702.

Tec, L. (1974). Nandrolone in anorexia nervosa (letter). *J. Amer. med. Assoc.* **229**, 1423.

Theander, S. (1970). Anorexia Nervosa. A psychiatric investigation of 94 female cases. *Acta psychiatr. scand.*, Suppl. 214, 1–194.

Thoma, H. (1967). "Anorexia Nervosa", International Universities Press, New York.

Vigersky, R. A. and Loriaux, D. L. (1977). The effect of cyproheptadine in anorexia nervosa: a double blind trial. *In* "Anorexia Nervosa" (R. A. Vigersky, ed.), pp. 349–356. Raven Press, New York.

Wakeling, A. and Russell, G. F. M. (1970). Disturbances in the regulation of body temperature in anorexia nervosa. *Psychol. Med.* **1**, 30–39.

Wakeling, A., Marshall, J. C., Beardwood, C. J., de Souza, V. F. A. and Russell, G. F. M. (1976). The effects of clomiphene citrate on the hypothalamic-pituitary gonadal axis in anorexia nervosa. *Psychol. Med.* **6**, 371–380.

Wakeling, A., de Souza, V. and Beardwood, C. J. (1977). Effects of administered oestrogen on luteinizing hormone release in subjects with anorexia nervosa in acute and recovery stages. *In* "Anorexia Nervosa" (R. A. Vigersky, ed.), pp. 199–210, Raven Press, New York.

Wakeling, A., De. Souza, V. F. A., Gore, M. B. R., Sabur, M., Kingstone, D. and Boss, A. M. B. (1979). Amenorrhoea, body weight and serum hormone concentrations with particular reference to prolactin and thyroid hormones in anorexia nervosa. *Psychol. Med.* **9**, 265–272.

Warren, M. P., and van de Wiele, R. L. (1973). Clinical and metabolic features of anorexia nervosa. *Amer. J. Obstet. Gynaec.* **117**, 435–449.

Williams, P. (1977). Anorexia Nervosa and the secretion of prolactin. *Brit. J. Psychiat.* **131**, 69–72.

Wirdum, P. van and Waber, A. (1961). The occurences of food preferences and aversions in groups of patients with peptic ulcer, asthma and neurosis. *J. Psychosom. Res.* **5**, 280.

Wurtman, R. J. and Fernstrom, J. D. (1976). Control of brain neurotransmitter synthesis by precursor availability and nutritional state. *Biochem. Pharm.* **25**, 1691–1696.

Yoshimoto, Y., Moridera, K. and Imara, H. (1975). Restoration of normal pituitary gonadotrophin reserve by administration of luteinizing hormone releasing hormone in patients with hypogonadotropic hypogonadism. *New Engl. J. Med.* **292**, 242–245.

Young, J. K. (1975). A possible neuroendocrine basis of two clinical syndromes: anorexia nervosa and the Klein-Levin syndrome. *Physiol. Psychol.* **3**, 322–330.

# ☐ Index

## A